# Deciphering the Dynamics of Hair Textures

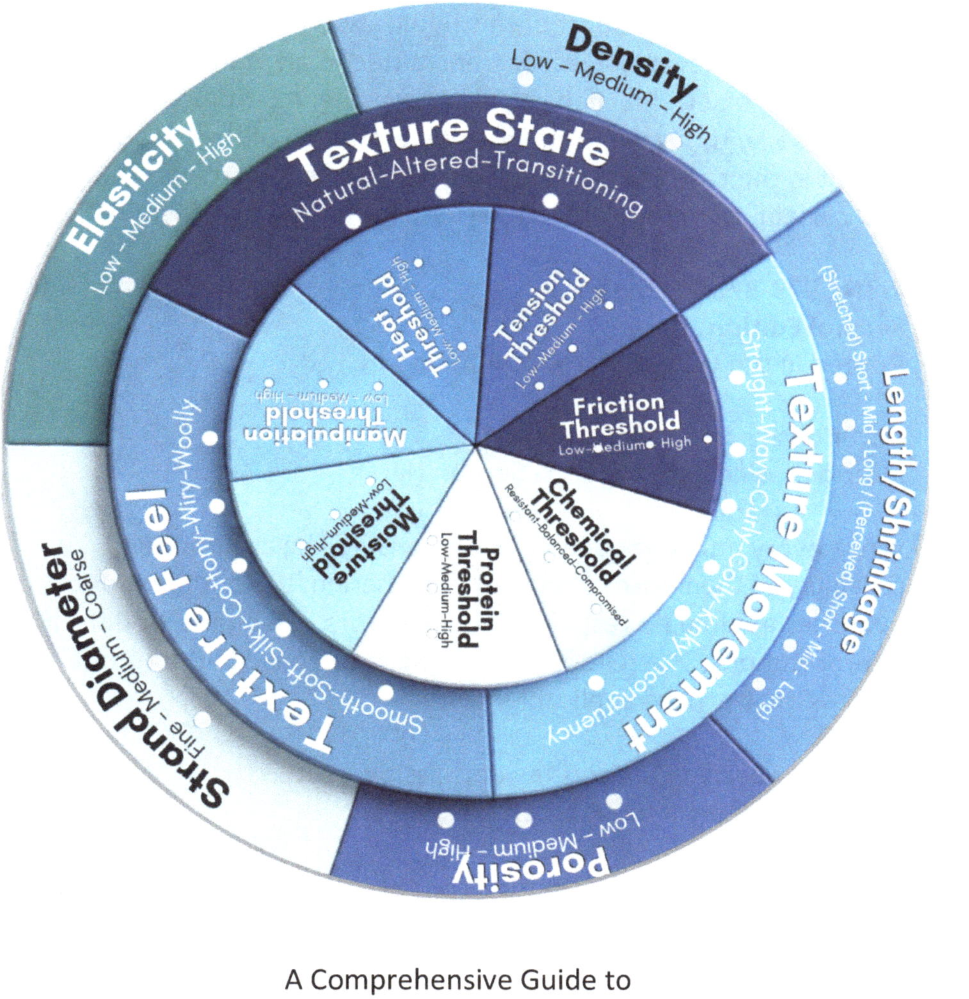

Density
Low - Medium - High

Texture State
Natural-Altered-Transitioning

Elasticity
Low - Medium - High

Length/Shrinkage
(Stretched) Short - Mid - Long / (Perceived) Short - Mid - Long)

Texture Movement
Straight-Wavy-Curly-Coily-Kinky-Incongruency

Porosity
Low - Medium - High

Strand Diameter
Fine - Medium - Coarse

Texture Feel
Smooth-Soft-Silky-Cottony-Wiry-Woolly

Heat Threshold
Low - Medium - High

Tension Threshold
Low - Medium - High

Friction Threshold
Low-Medium-High

Chemical Threshold
Resistant-Balanced-Compromised

Protein Threshold
Low-Medium-High

Moisture Threshold
Low-Medium-High

Manipulation Threshold
Low - Medium - High

A Comprehensive Guide to
Mastering the Science and Art of Hair Texture
Presented through the Texture Dynamics Framework™
2026 Edition

**Serriah L. Hart**

***Deciphering the Dynamics of Hair Texture*, 2026 Edition**
*Originally published as Deciphering the Dynamics of Textured Hair (2025)*



**ISBN:** 979-8-9925662-2-2
**Second Edition**
Printed in the United States of America

Cover design by Serriah Hart
Interior design and layout by Serriah Hart

While every effort has been made to ensure the accuracy and reliability of the information contained herein, the author and publisher assume no responsibility for errors, omissions, or differing interpretations. The reader is encouraged to consult appropriate professionals where applicable.

For more Learning & Licensing Permission, visit:
www.TextureDynamicsFramework.com

**Note to Reader:** The information contained in this book is provided for educational purposes only. While every effort has been made to ensure accuracy, the author and publisher make no representations or warranties of any kind, express or implied, regarding the completeness, accuracy, or applicability of the content herein. The author and publisher shall not be liable for any loss, injury, or damage arising from the use or misuse of information contained in this publication. Readers are advised to consult a licensed professional for specific applications.

## TABLE OF CONTENTS

**decipher**

de·ci·pher

1. to make out the meaning of despite indistinctness or obscurity
2. to interpret the meaning of

**dynamics**

dy·nam·ics

1. a pattern or process of change, growth, or activity
2. variation and contrast in force or intensity

**texture**

tex·ture

1 the visual or tactile surface characteristics and appearance of something

2. something composed of closely interwoven elements

# Introduction

For centuries, the beauty industry has centered straight hair as the systemic default for what was considered professional, beautiful, and desirable, keeping the industry stagnant and limiting its ability to evolve. In recent years, the term “Textured Hair” has narrowed its meaning to refer to variations of curls, causing confusion amid a series of oversimplified industry tropes. These assumptions didn't just shape product shelves and salon menus. It shaped curricula. It shaped the language professionals used when communicating with their clients. It shaped what consumers were taught to want from their own hair. This resulted in restricted exploration, the dismissal of a wide spectrum of natural expressions of beauty, and the beauty industry remaining comfortable in ignorance.

Today, that foundation is collapsing. And it should.

A global awakening, fueled by cultural pride, consumer awareness, and undeniable economic power, has forced the industry to confront what “Textured Hair” communities have always known: waves, coils, and curls are not niche. They are a cornerstone of global beauty. Coils, curls, kinks, waves, incongruent, and every movement in between represent billions of dollars in purchasing power and an even greater wealth of identity, story, and lived experience that the industry spent decades pretending didn't exist. And straight hair, as an aspect of hair texture rather than a standard of hair care, is now the reality.

Representation is increasing. Visibility is expanding. But visibility without understanding is not enough.

Because here is the truth, the industry has been slow to reckon with: most of the education driving hair schools, product marketing, and professional training today still relies on outdated, overly simplified, and dangerously narrow terminology, ignoring the complex behaviors that truly define it. These shallow systems cannot account for the real-life variations stylists encounter behind the chair, or consumers face in their bathroom sinks.

Existing industry language is ill-equipped to do the work of providing effective hair-texture fluency.

In over 27 years of working alongside some of the most skilled and passionate professionals this industry has produced, I saw a pattern that I could not look away from. Stylists were not avoiding certain hair textures because they didn't care. They were avoiding it because they had never been properly equipped to serve it. "Too difficult." "Too unpredictable." "Too time-consuming." I heard these words again and again, not as confessions of laziness, but as evidence of a system that had failed the people it was supposed to prepare.

As a Board-Certified Cosmetology Instructor, I watched curricula that centered almost entirely on how to straighten, relax, cover, or chemically alter hair texture. Rarely, almost never, on how to *understand* it in its natural state. The resources available to professionals were designed to control texture, not to decode it. And without decoding it, mastery was never possible.

I also watched consumers struggle on the other side of the same gap. Trying to find themselves in categories that weren't built around their experience. Reaching for products that presented an image for them to try to shrink their hair characteristics into. The industry was speaking a shorthand. Consumers were lost in translation. And no shared language existed to bridge the two.

*"Deciphering the Dynamics of Hair Textures"* exists to build that bridge.

This book does not provide a one-sided message of how to tame tight-textured hair. It teaches how to identify hair characteristics, potentials, and needs by understanding its structure, presentation, behavior, and limits. Inside, you will learn the Texture Dynamics Framework™: a tri-layered diagnostic system built on three pillars, Hair Properties, Texture Indicators™, and Hair Thresholds™. Together, they give you the most complete picture of how hair textures are built, how they move across the full Texture Movement Spectrum™, and how they respond under real-world conditions. Not as a category. But as a customized profile.

This is not a curl typing system with a new name. It is a language, precise, observable, and measurable, that allows stylists to consult with confidence, educators to teach what schools have never covered, brands to connect with the consumers they have been missing, and individuals to finally understand the hair they live with every single day.

This is not just a manual. It is a mindset shift.

Whether you are a stylist behind the chair, an educator in the classroom, a product developer in the lab, or someone standing in front of a mirror trying to make sense of your own crown, this book was written for you. Return to it. Argue with it. Let it challenge what you think you already know and replace assumptions with clarity.

The future of beauty is textured. And together, we’re shaping it!

If you have invested in this book, you’re ready to not just witness this paradigm shift, but to lead it. Here, leading means owning your craft with the kind of clarity that doesn't come from trends or tropes; it comes from understanding. It means being a problem solver who works from measurable data, not from assumptions, guesswork, or generalizations. It means teaching with precision instead of recycling the industry's oldest assumptions. It means building brands that speak to individual needs rather than echoing a collective shorthand that was never accurate to begin with. It means elevating what happens behind the chair and at the bathroom sink, because mastery at both levels is what permanently changes the experience of all hair textures.

You are at the beginning of that trajectory. And everything from here is elevation.

# 1.
# Modern History of Textured Hair Care

*From the Hot Comb to the Digital Age*

To truly decipher the dynamics of textured hair, we must first understand the historical forces that shaped how it has been perceived, studied, and taught. The history of textured hair care is simultaneously a cultural narrative, a scientific discipline, and an evolving commercial landscape, each dimension inseparable from the others. The same hair strand that carries identity and heritage also carries a chemistry that science is still refining and that the market has sought to understand and serve. To understand textured hair fully is to hold all of these truths at once. From the click of a hot comb on an early-1900s stovetop to the vibrant scroll of a natural hair tutorial on a smartphone screen, the journey of textured hair care is one of the most compelling and underexplored narratives in American social history.

What began as a conversation within the African American community has rippled outward, reshaping global beauty standards and inspiring people with highly textured hair on every continent to reclaim, celebrate, and care for. The evolution of curl care philosophies reflects nothing less than the long arc of a people's relationship with themselves.

This chapter traces this journey through its major eras, movements, innovators, and systems, from the pioneering entrepreneurs of the early nineteenth century to the digital-age educators and framework builders of today.

## The Era of Assimilation (1800s–1950s)

The story of modern textured hair care can be marked when enslaved Africans were forced onto the shores of America, the ceremonial and communal practices of hair care they had carried from their homelands were systematically stripped away, along with the natural ingredients, the time, the privacy, and the cultural context that had given those practices meaning. Without access to the butters, oils, and botanical preparations that had long been used to cleanse, condition, and protect their hair, enslaved people adapted with what was available. Lard and other household fats became substitutes for lost traditions. Plaits, cornrows, and head-tied scarves became both a protective necessity and a quiet cultural continuity, a way of keeping dignity and identity under conditions designed to erase both.

Meanwhile, a different standard was taking shape in the broader social landscape. Those who were not enslaved, and those whose hair fell into wavier or curlier, rather than tightly coiled patterns, understood early that texture carried social currency. Straighter, smoother hair was equated with refinement and respectability. Textured hair was straightened, pinned up, or curls were set. Any visible texture was carefully managed away. The hierarchy was not incidental. It was structural, a reflection of a society in which proximity to whiteness, in appearance as in all things, determined one's access to safety, opportunity, and dignity.

It was into this landscape that the early decades of the twentieth century arrived, and with them, the first formal industry built around the negotiation between Black hair and a world that had already decided what hair should look like.

### *The Birth of an Industry*

The heated metal pressing comb, commonly known as the hot comb, evolved from the Marcel iron, invented in 1872 by **Marcel Grateau**, a French hairdresser who revolutionized thermal hairstyling, and became a staple in African American households and beauty salons in this era. Pressed against a stovetop flame and drawn through tightly coiled strands, it temporarily straightened natural hair, conforming to the dominant aesthetic of the day. The ritual of the hot comb was simultaneously intimate and political: a weekly practice that produced sleek, straight styles considered more "presentable" in white-dominated professional and social spaces.

No figure looms larger over early Black hair care entrepreneurship than Sarah Breedlove, known to history as **Madame C.J. Walker** (1867–1919). Born to formerly enslaved parents in Louisiana, Walker developed and marketed a line of hair care products specifically formulated for Black women's hair, including her celebrated "Wonderful Hair Grower." Her system, encompassing products, techniques, and trained beauty agents, made her one of the first self-made female millionaires in American history. Madam C.J. Walker also popularized the hot comb in the early 1900s for African American hair. And **Walter Sammons,** a Black inventor from Philadelphia, later patented a significant improvement on the tool in 1920.

While Walker's products included straightening preparations, her broader mission was one of economic empowerment and hygiene education for Black women who had been historically excluded from mainstream beauty culture. She built a network of thousands of agents across the country, training Black women as professional beauticians and creating an early model of community-based commerce.

Simultaneously, hair relaxers, formulated to permanently straighten curly or kinky hair, originated between 1903-1913, when inventor **Garrett Augustus Morgan** accidentally discovered that an alkaline liquid designed to lubricate sewing machine needles also straightened wool, leading to the first chemical hair-refining cream. Chemical relaxers could permanently restructure the protein bonds in tightly textured hair and became an alternative to the hot comb. These products, while effective, came with significant risks: chemical burns, scalp damage, and long-term hair breakage. Yet for millions, they represented access to a professional world that privileged straight-haired appearances. The desire to straighten was rarely simply vanity; it was a survival strategy in a deeply unequal society. In the 1950s, **George E. Johnson** introduced "Ultra Sheen," a lye-based (sodium hydroxide) relaxer, which became a staple. By the 1970s, "no-lye" (guanidine hydroxide) options became popular to reduce scalp burns and damage. As early as the 1970s, concerns arose regarding scalp burns and hair loss, leading to mandatory warning labels by 1975. In recent years, scientific studies have linked the long-term use of these products to health issues such as uterine and breast cancer, sparking thousands of lawsuits. This has created a major shift away from chemical relaxers, with many women transitioning back to their natural textures, reversing the long-standing cultural norm of chemically straightened hair.

Beyond the Black American experience, the curly perm originated in 1905 when German hairdresser **Karl Nessler** introduced a six-hour heat-based machine to create long-lasting curls. The process evolved from risky early-20th-century electric, chemical-based heating methods to the safe "cold waves" of the 1940s, eventually peaking in popularity with the big, tight, curly styles of the 1980s.

## Rise of the Afro – First Wave of The Natural Hair Movement (1960s–1970s)

If the early twentieth century was defined by the need to assimilate textured hair, the 1960s marked an explosive and deliberate cultural reversal. The Civil Rights Movement did not simply demand political equality; it demanded a total reimagining of Black identity, dignity, and beauty.

The Afro, a rounded, voluminous style that allows natural coils to expand freely from the scalp without chemical alteration, heat, or suppression, became the defining aesthetic emblem of an era. It was not a style that emerged by sheer fashion trend. It was chosen by a generation that had grown up watching their mothers press, relax, and pin their natural texture into socially acceptable submission. The decision to wear the hair as it grew was a political act as deliberate as a sit-in or a march.

Rooted in the "Black Is Beautiful" movement, wearing an Afro was a deliberate act of defiance against Eurocentric beauty standards that had long deemed natural Black hair "unkempt," "professionally inappropriate," or simply inferior. To wear the Afro was to refuse assimilation on those terms. Afro care products began to bloom, and a new niche was born.

No image crystallized this more powerfully than that of Angela Davis. A scholar, activist, and Communist Party member, Davis became one of the most photographed and circulated faces of Black radical politics in the early 1970s. Her large, perfectly symmetrical Afro appeared on FBI wanted posters, protest flyers, newspaper front pages, and magazine covers across the world, and in doing so, transformed a hairstyle into an international symbol. To see the Afro was to see resistance. Governments and institutions that sought to suppress Black political organizing found themselves unable to separate the politics from the hair. In some schools and workplaces, the Afro was explicitly banned, a response that only confirmed what its wearers already knew: that the hair was never simply hair.

The period also witnessed a broader reclamation of styles rooted in African heritage and tradition. Cornrows, once suppressed as markers of enslavement and poverty, were reframed as expressions of artistry and cultural lineage. Locs, comb coils, and other natural styles that had existed in African communities for centuries found new visibility and new meaning in the American context, no longer signs of otherness to be overcome, but evidence of a rich and unbroken heritage to be worn with pride.

It was also during this period that the first commercial infrastructure around natural Black hair began to take shape. Afro care products, picks, natural oils, sheen sprays, and moisturizers formulated for unprocessed texture, began appearing on shelves, marking the first time the market had moved toward natural hair rather than away from it.

## From Jheri Curls to Natural Salons – Second Wave of The Natural Hair Movement (1980s–1990s)

As the political energy of the 1960s gave way to the more commercially driven culture of the 1980s, the Afro receded from its dominant cultural position. In its place emerged styles that blended natural texture with chemical enhancement, most notably, the Jheri curl.

Invented by hair care entrepreneur **Jheri Redding** and popularized through the 1980s, the Jheri curl used a two-step chemical process to create soft, glossy, loose ringlets. The style dominated Black popular culture, from entertainers to professionals.

Simultaneously, synthetic braid extensions experienced a sudden boom as Cornrows, box braids, Senegalese twists, and other styles rooted in African tradition gained renewed visibility and sophistication with the growing availability of synthetic braiding hair. By the late 1990s, Black braiding professionals were at the center of regulatory battles in multiple U.S. states, fighting for the right to practice their craft without state-mandated cosmetology licenses that were designed around European hair types, an early legal skirmish in what would become an ongoing struggle for professional recognition of textured hair expertise.

Natural Hair Salons became a pivotal source of proper hair care for highly textured hair. This period witnessed the rise of braids, locs, comb coils, and other protective styles drawn from African traditions, all reframed as expressions of cultural pride, creativity, and beauty.

The 1980s and 1990s had produced a textured hair landscape of remarkable variety and contradiction: chemical curls sitting alongside protective styles, relaxers alongside locs, mainstream entertainment aesthetics alongside growing Afrocentric pride. Consumers, stylists, and product developers were working across this spectrum without a shared framework for understanding what they were working with. It was into this gap that André Walker stepped.

## The History of Black Hair Education: From African Roots to Professional Discipline

The history of Black hair education did not begin in classrooms or formal institutions. It began within the cultural, spiritual, and social systems of African civilizations, where hair functioned as a powerful form of communication. Across many West African societies, hairstyles conveyed identity, lineage, age, marital status, religion, and social position. Hair was not merely styled, it was understood. It was a living language, taught through observation, participation, and generational transfer.

This deeply rooted system of knowledge was violently disrupted during the transatlantic slave trade. Enslaved Africans were stripped of their cultural identity upon arrival, often having their heads shaved as a deliberate act of humiliation and control. This act symbolized more than physical loss. It severed a direct connection to heritage, status, and self-expression.

Despite these conditions, Black communities found ways to preserve elements of their traditions. Hair care became an act of resistance and survival. Techniques such as braiding, the use of natural herbs, and communal grooming practices were passed down informally. Education existed without formal recognition, sustained through shared experience and cultural memory.

During the colonial period, particularly in Louisiana, hair remained a site of both oppression and expression. The Tignon Laws of 1786 required women of African descent to cover their hair in public as a marker of social inferiority. Rather than submit to erasure, these women transformed the mandate into a form of artistry. Headwraps were styled with intention, creativity, and elegance, preserving cultural pride in the face of restriction. What was meant to diminish identity instead reinforced it.

Following the abolition of slavery, Black hair continued to be judged against Eurocentric beauty standards. Textures that deviated from these ideals were stigmatized, creating both social and economic barriers. This environment led to a growing need for structured education, product development, and economic independence within Black communities.

In the early 20th century, this need gave rise to the formalization of Black hair education. Pioneers such as Annie Turnbo Malone established institutions like Poro College, one of the first comprehensive centers dedicated to Black cosmetology. These institutions were not simply beauty schools. They were hubs of education, entrepreneurship, and empowerment, providing training in hair care, business, and self-sufficiency.

Madam C.J. Walker expanded this model by developing a national network of trained professionals, often referred to as "hair culturists." Through her educational programs and distribution systems, thousands of Black women gained access to financial independence and professional skill development. Hair education became both a craft and a pathway to economic mobility.

By the mid-20th century, cosmetology became regulated across the United States. However, segregation limited access to education and professional opportunities for Black cosmetologists, particularly in the South. In response, Black educators and entrepreneurs continued to build their own institutions and advocacy organizations, ensuring that Black hair care remained both studied and protected. Events such as the Bronner Bros. Trade Show, founded in Atlanta in 1947, played a significant role in advancing professional education. These gatherings created spaces for learning, innovation, and community, elevating Black hair care into a recognized and evolving discipline.

In more recent decades, the natural hair movement has further expanded the scope of Black hair education. Leaders in the space have created platforms, shows, and training systems dedicated specifically to natural textures, braiding, and holistic hair care. One of the first to offer braiding classes on a large scale was Taliah Waajid, best known as the founder of the World Natural Hair Show, the world's largest, longest-running, Black-owned, and operated event focused on natural hair, culture, health, and beauty. These efforts have re-centered textured hair as something to be understood, not altered.

Today, Black hair education exists at the intersection of culture, science, and professional practice. It has evolved from ancestral knowledge systems into a structured industry, yet its foundation remains the same. It is rooted in identity, adaptation, and resilience. Understanding this history is essential. It reveals that Black hair education has never been simply about styling. It has always been about knowledge, preservation, and the power to define beauty on one's own terms.

### *The Andre Walker Typing System*

It was against this backdrop of growing commercial and cultural complexity that celebrity stylist **André Walker**, best known as Oprah Winfrey's personal hairdresser, introduced what would become the most widely used hair classification system in modern history. Developed in the 1990s to market his line of hair care products, Walker's system organized all human hair into four main categories based on curl pattern and texture.

| Type | Category | Characteristics |
| --- | --- | --- |
| Type 1 A-C | Straight | Fine & Fragile to Coarse & Thin (Curl Resistant) |
| Type 2 A-C | Wavy | Fine & Thin to Coarse & Frizzy |
| Type 3 A-C | Curly | Loose Curls & Corkscrew Curls |
| Type 4 A-C | Coily / Kinky | Tight Coils to Z-Angled Coils |

Walker's system gained its greatest public platform through the Oprah Winfrey Show, where it was introduced to a mainstream audience and rapidly adopted by salons, beauty bloggers, and product developers across the country. The 1A-4C classification became the shared vocabulary that allowed individuals to seek out products, techniques, and tutorials specifically suited to their curl pattern.

From the outset, the system attracted both enthusiastic adoption and pointed criticism. Proponents valued its practical utility: knowing your "hair type" could predict how products would absorb, how chemical treatments would react, and which styling methods would yield the best results. Critics, however, argued that the system was fundamentally a marketing framework rather than a scientific one, and that it introduced a subtle hierarchy that privileged looser curl patterns (3A–3C) over the tightly coiled 4-type textures that are most common among people of West and Central African descent, inadvertently reproduced, in encoded form, the colorist and texture biases it claimed to neutralize.

Despite these critiques, the Walker system remains the dominant reference point in curl care discourse, and its adoption marked a pivotal moment: the beginning of a systematic, analytical approach to textured hair that would be refined and expanded by a new generation of innovators in the years to come.

**The Curly Girl Method**

While the Walker system provided a language for describing textured hair, a parallel revolution was underway in New York City's salon culture. Hairstylist and author **Lorraine Massey**, working with clients whose curly hair had been repeatedly damaged by conventional salon practices, began developing a radical alternative philosophy, one that would ultimately reach millions of people around the world.

Massey, a British-born stylist who emigrated to the United States, drew on her own experience with wavy hair and her observations of countless clients to begin formulating what she called the Curly Girl Method (CGM): a philosophy of working with textured hair's natural structure rather than against it.

The method was formally introduced to a global audience in her 2001 book, *Curly Girl: The Handbook*, co-written with Deborah Chiel. The book offered a comprehensive alternative to conventional hair care by establishing a strict set of guidelines designed to protect and restore the hair cuticle:

- **No Shampoo** (Co-Washing, a practice that the Natural Hair Community had been using as a refresher between wash days, rather than a replacement for wash days)
- **No silicone-containing products**
- **No Heat Styling**
- **No Brushes or Combs**
- **No Harmful ingredients:** drying alcohols, certain synthetic fragrances,
- **Become active readers of ingredient lists**, a practice that would fundamentally reshape how consumers engage with beauty products.

The CGM also reframed the concept of the 'Wash and Go', a term that had entered mainstream beauty vocabulary through Vidal Sassoon's 1987 UK product line, where it simply meant a quick, low-effort routine for manageable, straight-leaning hair. Massey reclaimed and redefined the term entirely, repositioning it as a philosophy of curl liberation: apply products to soaking-wet hair, allow it to air-dry in its natural state, and trust the curl to do what it was always designed to do. Techniques like plopping and scrunching, both designed to encourage curl formation rather than suppress it, became central to the method. In Massey's hands, 'Wash and Go' was no longer a convenience pitch, it was a declaration that natural texture required no correction. Massey presented the term as a method that involves applying products to soaking-wet hair and allowing it to air-dry, typically focusing on conditioner rather than shampoo. Techniques often include "plopping" and "scrunching" to define curls.

Massey also developed a specialized cutting technique, the Deva Cut, which involved cutting curly hair dry, strand by strand, in its natural curl state rather than wet and stretched as was conventional practice. The Deva Cut allowed stylists to see and shape the hair as it actually lived and moved, rather than guessing at how it would behave once dry. It became one of the foundational techniques of the modern natural hair salon.

## Digital Natural Hair Movement– Third Wave of The Natural Hair Movement (2000s–Present)

The 2000s brought a convergence of forces that would ignite the most powerful revival of natural hair culture in American history. A rising generation of African American women, armed with the internet and motivated by deepening critiques of Eurocentric beauty standards and a need for healthy hair care options, began sharing their natural hair journeys online, and the movement they built would eventually reshape a global industry.

### *Online Communities and the Big Chop*

Forums like NaturallyCurly.com, BlackHairMedia, and later YouTube channels, Facebook, and Instagram accounts created unprecedented spaces for Black women to discuss their hair on their own terms. The act of "transitioning", gradually growing out chemically relaxed hair, or the more dramatic "big chop" (cutting all chemically processed hair at once to start fresh with natural growth) became shared rituals, documented in photographs and videos that circulated virally through these communities.

What the digital age made possible was not just community, it was accountability and collective knowledge-building. Women shared what worked and what didn't. They analyzed ingredient lists, filmed step-by-step tutorials, and debated the merits of various techniques across thousands of comment threads.

Styling trends like stretched styles, twist-and-tuck pinned styles, two-strand twists, twist-outs, braid-outs, and other creative ways of styling highly textured hair in its natural state became sought-after content. However, there was a gap between hair inspiration and availability for products that catered to the needs of textured hair.

### *The Rise of Black-Owned Natural Hair Brands*

The natural hair movement created both demand and opportunity. Entrepreneurs recognized that the major cosmetics corporations had long neglected the specific needs of textured hair, and moved to fill the gap. Companies like Carol's Daughter (founded by **Lisa Price** in Brooklyn, New York in 1993 from a kitchen pot) emerged as pioneering examples of Black-owned brands built specifically around natural, textured hair care. Price's products, centered on natural ingredients and moisture retention, became emblematic of a new kind of beauty company: one that treated natural hair as something to be nourished rather than corrected.

The 2010s saw an explosion of such brands as Shea Moisture brand, founded by Richelieu Dennis in 1991 in Harlem, Camille Rose, Mielle Organics, Aunt Jackie's, and dozens of others, creating a multi-billion-dollar industry segment that had not existed a generation before. These brands were more than commercial enterprises; they were cultural declarations, each product formulation a statement about what textured hair deserved.

The natural hair movement also fueled a broader political reckoning. The passage of **CROWN Act legislation** (Creating a Respectful and Open World for Natural Hair) in multiple U.S. states beginning in 2019 made it illegal to discriminate against individuals based on their natural hair texture or protective styles in workplaces and schools, a legal recognition that natural hair had long been used as a pretext for racial discrimination.

## Evolution of the Wash and Go to Curl Definition.

The community knowledge sharing within the Digital Natural Hair Movement spread the philosophies of the Curly Girl Method far beyond the book's reach. This led the Natural hair community to take on and redefine terms like "wash and go" and "co-wash" in an attempt to live in their free, natural curl pattern. Miss Jessie's, founded by **Miko and Titi Branch**, began developing their signature styling techniques, including the shingling method, around 1999–2004, coinciding with the opening of their salon and the launch of their product line to serve the natural curly hair market. The technique was designed to define curls, especially using Miss Jessie's Curly Pudding.

As the Digital Natural Hair Movement matured, a gap became increasingly visible between the inspiration the community was generating online and the practical reality for those with the tightest textures. The mainstream Wash and Go, as presented across digital platforms, consistently delivered defined, bouncy results for wavier and loosely curly hair types. For those with "Type 4 coils and zig-zag patterns", however, the same techniques rarely translated, and the products' promised definition was not designed with their texture in mind.

It was into this gap that curl specialist, educator, and Curl Definition brand founder, Serriah Hart, stepped in with a methodical and technique-driven response. In 2013, Hart introduced the Curl Definition Method, a technique specifically developed to define highly textured hair using a three-row Curl Defining comb. Rather than relying on the product alone to encourage curl formation. The prevailing approach of the Wash and Go, Hart's method physically guided the tighter curl into ringlets, creating defined curl formations through intentional, precise manipulation. The technique represented a meaningful departure from the assumption that all curl patterns would respond the same way to the same approach. To share and demonstrate the method directly with the professional community, Hart began hosting hair shows in New York.

In 2015, Hart expanded her work by introducing the Curl Training System and simultaneously launching the Curl Definition product line. The system introduced the concept of Curl Training, which understands hair as a fiber with memory, capable of being guided over time to respond more predictably and consistently to definition, moisture, and manipulation. Where most curl care approaches addressed the hair as it presented on any given wash day, the Curl Training System offered something more ambitious: a sustained, progressive methodology that, practiced consistently over months, could fundamentally shift how the hair behaved. It gave stylists and home practitioners alike not just a technique for a single good result, but a roadmap toward a transformed hair health trajectory. Hart began presenting at Bronner Brothers' Hair Show and the Talija Wajiid World Natural Hair Show, establishing herself as an educator and innovator within the natural hair space.

Hart's most comprehensive contribution came in 2018 with her Hair-acteristics class, which later developed into the Texture Dynamics Framework, formalized in 2021. The framework moved beyond both curl typing and training protocols to address the full ecology of textured hair, integrating hair properties, hair behaviors, and hair limitations into a unified analytical model. Where previous systems had tended to treat these variables in isolation, the Texture Dynamics Framework offered a holistic approach, a way to understand how each characteristic influences the others and how targeted interventions at any point in the system could assess and produce measurable improvements in overall hair health and appearance. Central to the framework is the Texture Profile Wheel, which provides consumers, educators, stylists, and brands with a precise and systematic tool for analyzing and communicating a multidimensional profile of hair beyond the limitations of curl typing and conventional hair analysis. It positioned textured hair care not as a niche beauty practice but as a discipline with its own rigorous and reproducible body of knowledge.

## Global Reach, A Movement Without Borders

The philosophies, frameworks, and cultural values generated by a century of Black American engagement with natural hair have traveled, through the internet, through diaspora networks, through global media, and through the quiet recognition of shared experience, to reach people with highly textured hair on every inhabited continent.

In Brazil, where people of African descent constitute the majority of the population and where a deeply entrenched colorist hierarchy has long stigmatized natural Black hair, the natural hair movement has gained powerful momentum. Brazilian natural hair activists have drawn explicitly on the language and frameworks of the American movement while developing their own distinctive political and aesthetic vocabulary, reclaiming the term "cabelo crespo" (kinky hair) as a source of pride rather than shame.

In West and East Africa, where natural textures had never been culturally stigmatized to the same degree, the global natural hair conversation has nonetheless introduced new frameworks, products, and techniques that have expanded the vocabulary of hair care for millions. The Walker typing system, CGM principles, and frameworks like Hart's Texture Dynamics have found audiences in Nigeria, Kenya, Ghana, South Africa, and beyond.

In Europe, particularly in France, the United Kingdom, and the Netherlands, countries with large Afro-descendant and mixed-heritage populations, the natural hair movement has become intertwined with broader struggles for racial equity and visibility. Natural hair YouTubers, bloggers, and educators in these countries have created thriving communities that draw on American frameworks while addressing the specific social and product availability challenges of their own contexts.

Even communities of mixed heritage in South and Southeast Asia, Latin America, and the Middle East, where wavy and loosely coiled textures are common but often poorly served by the beauty industry, have found resonance in the natural hair movement's core message: that textured hair, in all its forms, deserves care, knowledge, and celebration on its own terms.

The movement is not finished. There are still workplaces that discriminate, still beauty industries that underserve, still children who are told their hair is "too much." But the philosophical foundation has been laid, the vocabulary has been built, and the global community has been assembled. The crown, it turns out, was always there. The work, the beautiful, ongoing, transformative work, has been learning how to wear it.

# TEXTURE PROFILE WHEEL™

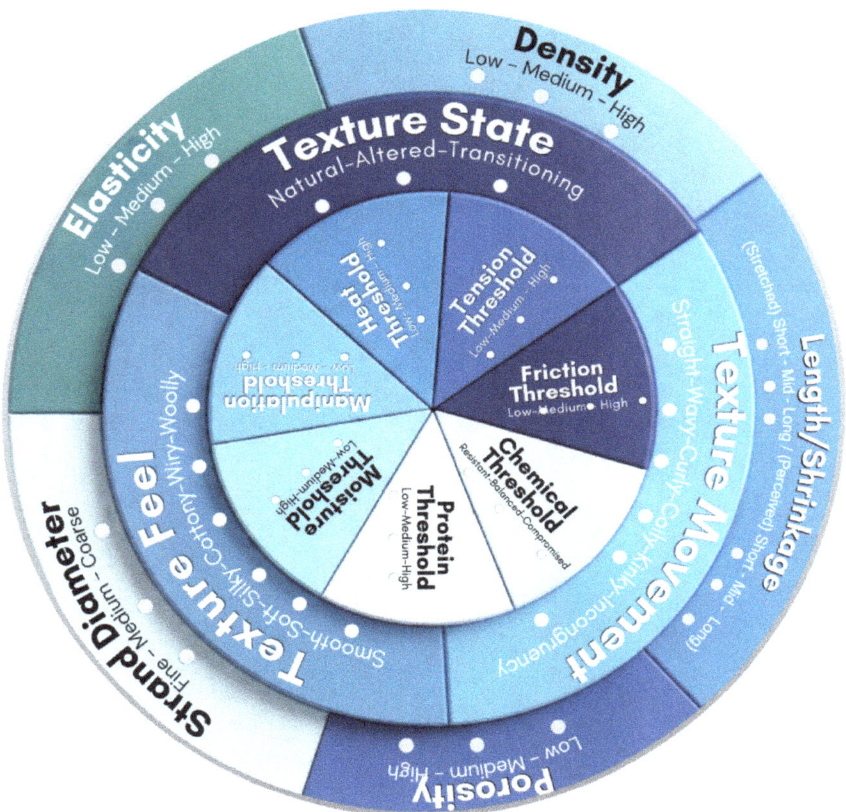


# TEXTURE MOVEMENT SPECTRUM™

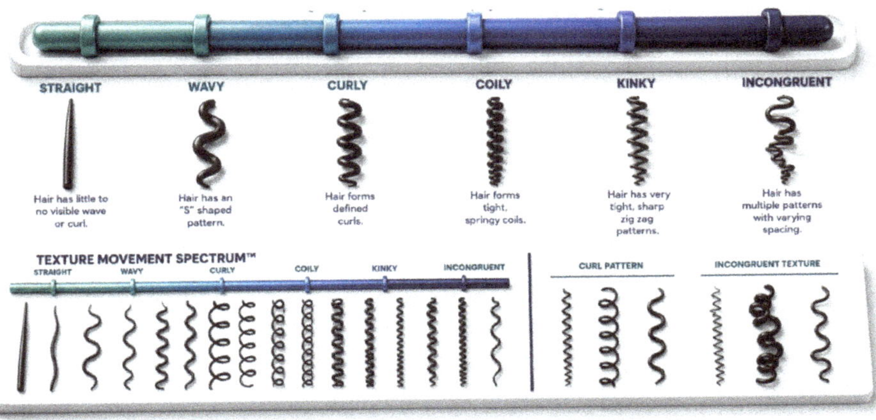

# 2.
# Texture Dynamics Framework™
*& Exploring Hair Anatomy*

## The Texture Dynamics Framework™ and Exploring Hair Anatomy

The history of textured hair education reveals a consistent pattern, one shaped by over-simplification, limitation, and a disconnect from the lived experience of textured hair. For decades, hair has been categorized through narrow systems that attempt to define it by a single characteristic, often reducing texture to curl pattern or strand diameter. While these systems provided a starting point, they have not fully equipped professionals or individuals to understand the true complexity of textured hair.

As a result, many are left navigating their hair through trial and error, relying on generalized advice that fails to account for the unique combination of traits that define each individual's texture. This gap between traditional education and real-world application highlights the need for something more comprehensive, more precise, and more adaptable.

To move forward, we must shift from simplified classifications to a deeper, more dynamic understanding of hair. This requires more than new terminology. It requires a structured system that allows us to observe, interpret, and respond to hair in a way that reflects its full complexity.

This is where the Texture Dynamics Framework™ comes in.

The **Texture Dynamics Framework™** is a modernized analytical methodology that expands traditional hair analysis into a more interconnected understanding of hair structure, presentation, behavior, thresholds, and response. Rather than viewing hair through isolated characteristics or rigid categories, TDF™ approaches hair as a dynamic texture identity spanning a full spectrum of texture expression, recognizing that every head exists as its own multidimensional texture profile.

At its core, the framework is 15 dimensions built into **Three Pillars of Hair™**:

- **Pillar 1 - Hair Properties™** – the structural and measurable characteristics of the hair, including elasticity, porosity, density, strand diameter, and length
- **Pillar 2 - Texture Indicators™** – how the hair presents visually and physically, including its shape, pattern, and tactile feel
- **Pillar 3 - Hair Thresholds™** – the limits and sensitivities that determine how the hair responds to moisture, protein, heat, manipulation, tension, and friction

Together, these pillars form the basis of a **Texture Profile™**, a personalized assessment that captures the full scope of an individual's hair characteristics. This profile serves as a guide to making informed decisions about product selection, styling techniques, maintenance routines, and long-term hair health. The **Texture Profile Wheel™** is a visual and diagnostic tool that presents a comprehensive representation of the 15 dimensions of hair in a snapshot of an individual's Texture Profile. The Texture Profile Wheel™ serves as the ultimate hair analysis tool, tracking the dynamic and multidimensional nature of each individual's hair, providing analysis that exceeds industry standards. By collectively assessing these characteristics, you gain a more tailored, comprehensive view of each client's hair care needs. This holistic approach transforms hair care from a one-size-fits-all practice into a truly personalized and professional art.

The Texture Dynamics Framework™ transforms hair care from a one-size-fits-all approach into a tailored, intentional practice. It provides a shared language for professionals, educators, and individuals, allowing for clearer communication, more accurate assessments, and more consistent results.

This book is designed to guide you through each component of this framework in a structured and progressive way. You will begin with **Pillar 1 - Hair Properties™**, where you will explore the internal structure of the hair and the measurable traits that define its foundation. From there, you will move into **Pillar 2 - Texture Indicators™**, gaining a deeper understanding of how hair presents and behaves in its natural and altered states. You will then examine **Pillar 3 - Hair Thresholds™**, learning how to identify the limits that influence how hair responds to products, styling, and environmental factors.

Beyond these pillars, this book introduces you to **Scalp Spatial Distribution™ (SSD)**, an advanced approach to mapping and working with the variation of hair characteristics across different areas of the scalp. You will also explore the **Aesthetics of Beauty**, helping you distinguish between enhancing natural traits and achieving desired visual outcomes. Finally, you will learn practical strategies for **Managing Textured Hair** by applying the principles of the framework in real-world scenarios.

Each chapter builds upon the last, creating a system that is both educational and actionable. As you move through this book, you are not just learning about hair; you are developing the ability to assess, interpret, and respond to it with precision and confidence.

Before we can fully apply this framework, however, we must first establish a clear understanding of what hair is at its most fundamental level.

## What is Hair

Let's start by establishing the foundation of what Hair is and, more specifically, "what is Textured Hair". **Hair** is a thread-like filament of dead, keratinized protein cells that grow from follicles in the scalp. Hair is composed of three layers. The outermost layer of the hair is the **Cuticle,** consisting of a single overlapping layer of transparent scale-like cells. The **Cortex** is the middle layer of the hair, containing melanin pigment and fibrous protein, and the **Medulla** is the innermost layer of the hair, composed of round cells containing mainly air space. The structure of the hair is made up of the **Hair Root,** which is enclosed within the follicle beneath the skin surface, the **Hair Shaft** that extends beyond the skin surface, the **Hair Follicle** that holds the hair root, and the **Hair Bulb** that forms the lower part of the hair root.

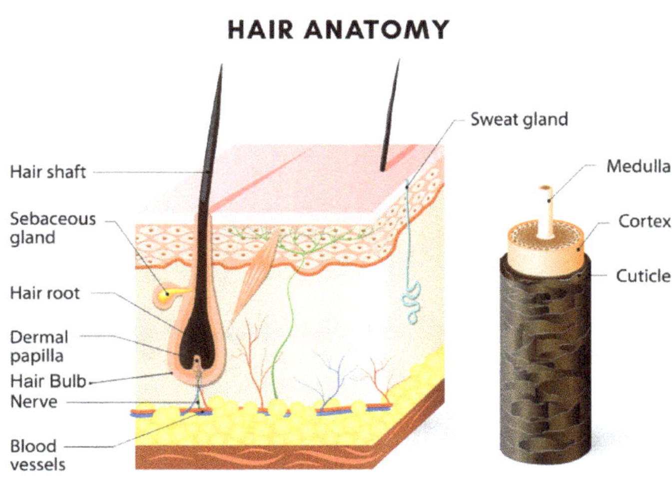


## Hair Bond Structure

Hair is made of a protein called keratin, which is like a string of tiny amino acid beads connected together, called polypeptide chains. These strings twist into coils and bunch up to make the inside of each hair strand. The coils are then connected by three types of bonds:

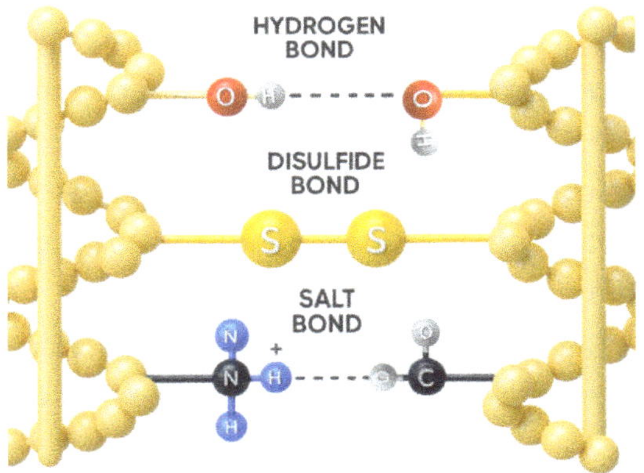


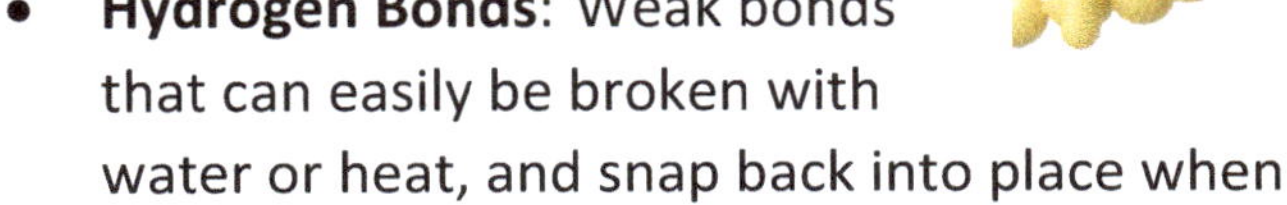

- **Hydrogen Bonds**: Weak bonds that can easily be broken with water or heat, and snap back into place when hair dries or cools.

- **Salt Bonds:** Bonds are formed between positive and negative charges, are easily broken by changes in pH, and reconnect once the pH balance is restored.
- **Disulfide Bonds:** Very strong bonds that can only be changed with chemicals like relaxers, perms, or bleach, or extreme heat. They're what give the hair shape.

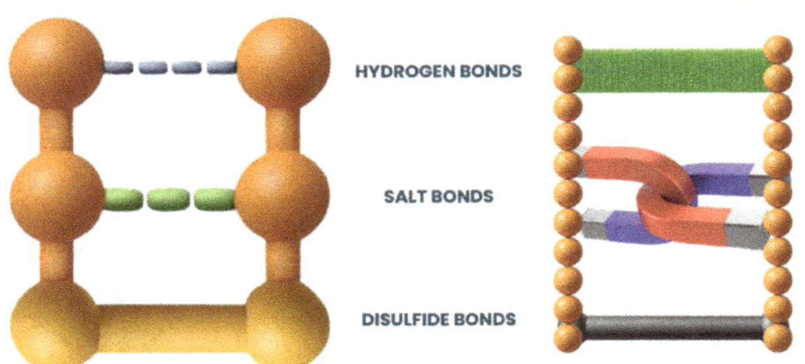


Together, these connections are what make hair strong, flexible, and able to hold its shape. Like the attachment of Velcro, Hydrogen bonds are easily broken and easily reattached. Similar to how magnets easily attract to the opposite charge and are broken when the attraction is interrupted, Salt Bonds are easily broken when the hair's pH changes (shampoo, conditioner, products), but reconnect when pH balance is restored. Just as the strong bond of a welded metal rod is very hard to break, the attachment of disulfide bonds is very hard to break, and can only be changed with chemicals or extreme heat.

## What is Hair Texture

In everyday applications, hair is described by its feel, appearance, or the consistency of its surface or substance. These descriptions match the real-world application of the phrase "texture of" as utilized in art textiles and even extend to describe music and sound. However, in contrast, conventional cosmetology standards narrow the definition of "texture" to refer only to the diameter of a hair strand. This definition overlooks the broader use of the term in both the professional beauty industry and tactile use. There is a need to bridge the industry gap between cosmetology standards and real-life applications. The term **Hair Texture™** is best defined as the overall appearance and tactile experience of hair, encompassing its shape, movement, and feel.

Traditional methods of hair analysis often focus on the basic properties of porosity, texture, elasticity, and density, and rely heavily on limited curl typing systems (e.g., 2A to 4C) to classify hair. While these systems provide a starting point, they are insufficient in fully addressing the complexity and diversity of hair characteristics. This limited approach shrinks broad ranges of unique hair traits into oversimplified categories, overlooking the nuanced differences that impact how hair responds to care, styling, and treatments.

The concept of texture extends far beyond the diameter of a hair strand; it is dynamic in nature and intertwined with almost every other hair property. The most effective way to analyze the dynamic characteristics of hair textures is to create a Texture Profile™, unique to each client. Developing a comprehensive texture profile expands hair analysis by considering the full spectrum of hair traits, including hair properties (elasticity, porosity, strand diameter, and length), texture indicators (shape, pattern, and feel), thresholds (protein, moisture, heat, manipulation, tension), and individual experiences (e.g., life-style, environmental exposure, cultural practices, and styling habits). This approach ensures that specific needs are met and avoids the risk of disregarding unique traits that fall outside conventional frameworks.

## Key Terms

**Texture Dynamics Framework™**: A comprehensive approach to identifying, understanding, and caring for an individual's unique hair traits by use of a personalized tri-layered assessment.

**Three Pillars of Hair Texture™**: Hair Properties, Texture Indicators, and Hair Thresholds.

**Texture Profile™:** a personalized assessment that captures the full scope of an individual's hair characteristics.

**Texture Profile Wheel™**: A hair analysis tool that evaluates the complexity of each individual's hair texture.

**Hair**: A thread-like filament of dead, keratinized protein cells that grow from follicles in the scalp.

**Cuticle:** The outermost layer of the hair.

**Cortex**: The middle layer of the hair, containing melanin pigment and fibrous protein.

**Medulla**: The innermost layer of the hair, composed of round cells containing mainly airspace.

**Hair Root**: The structure of the hair enclosed within the follicle beneath the skin surface.

**Hair Shaft**: The structure of the hair that extends beyond the skin surface.

**Hair Follicle**: The structure of the hair that holds the hair root.

**Hair Bulb**: The structure of the hair that forms the lower part of the hair root.

**Hydrogen Bonds**: Weak bonds that can easily be broken with water or heat.

**Salt Bonds**: Hair bonds formed between positive and negative charges that are easily broken by changes in pH.

**Disulfide Bonds**: Very strong bonds that can only be changed with chemicals like relaxers, perms, or bleach, or extreme heat.

**Hair Texture™**: The overall appearance and tactile experience of the hair, encompassing the shape, movement, and feel of the hair.

# Texture Dynamics - Pillar 1
# HAIR PROPERTIES™
## HAIR STRUCTURE

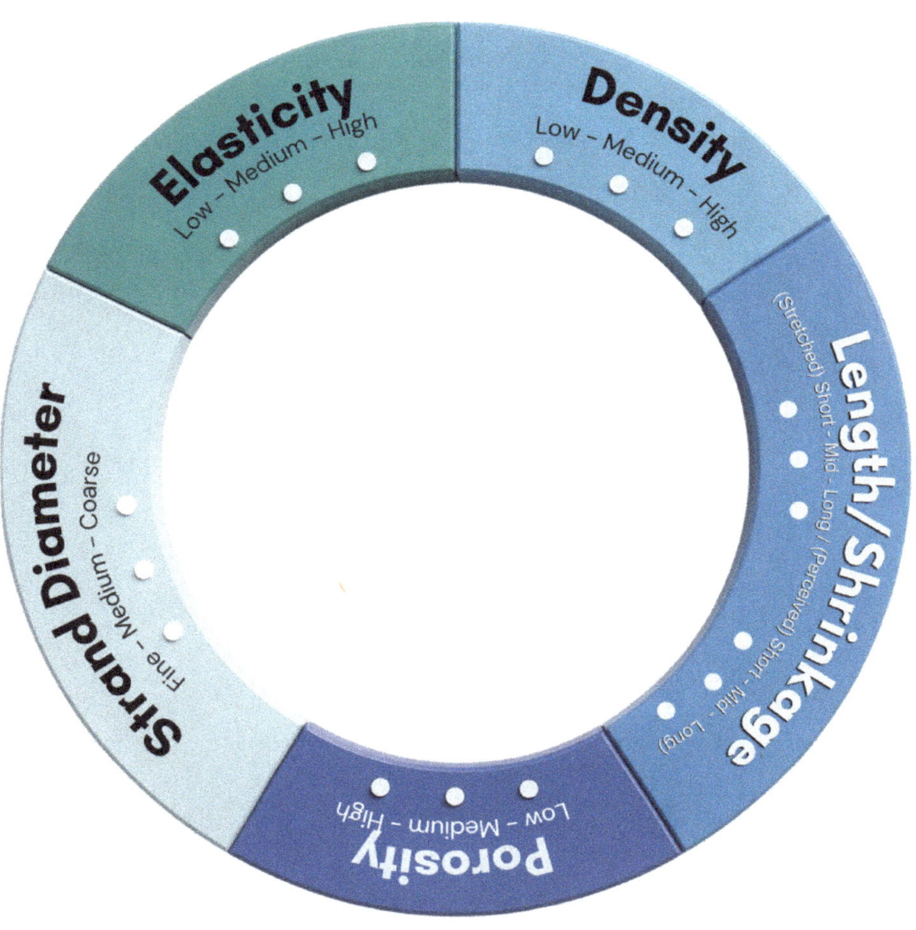

# 3.
# Pillar 1 - Hair Properties

*How Texture Is Structured*

The term **Hair Properties** refers to specific hair traits that determine hair's appearance, behavior, and overall health. The four main Hair Properties consist of:

- **Elasticity** – How much the hair can stretch without breaking, and return to its original shape.
- **Density** – The number of hair strands growing from the scalp per square inch and the number of follicles active on the scalp per square inch.
- **Length –** The measurement of hair from root to end.
- **Porosity –** Hair's ability to absorb, retain, and release moisture.
- **Strand Diameter** – The width of an individual strand of hair.

Understanding these hair properties enables professionals to tailor their services to each client's unique hair needs and identify how hair responds to different styling techniques, treatments, and products.

## Elasticity

Hair **Elasticity** refers to the hair's ability to stretch and return to its original shape without breaking. According to the National Library of Medicine, healthy hair can stretch up to 20–30% of its length when dry and as much as 50% when wet. This property is essential for hair health and is crucial for managing hair textures. To maintain optimal hair elasticity, it is important to achieve a healthy balance between moisture and protein levels in the hair.

The **Moisture Level™** in hair refers to the amount of water content within the hair strands. This directly affects the hair's manageability, elasticity, softness, flexibility, and pliability. The Moisture Level is determined by the hair's porosity (its ability to absorb and retain water) and its external environment, such as humidity and exposure to drying factors like heat or chemicals. Hair needs adequate moisture to maintain its structural integrity and prevent dryness, brittleness, and breakage. This moisturization begins by hydrating the hair with water, water-based products, or a hydrating treatment. The moisture absorbed affects hydrated hair's ability to stretch, temporarily enhancing its flexibility. Applying oil and emollient-based products to hydrated hair can help seal in this moisture, ensuring the hair remains pliable and less likely to snap under tension.

While moisture is essential, the overall tensile strength of the hair depends heavily on the cortex's keratin protein content. Without sufficient keratin, the elasticity provided by moisture retention becomes superficial and short-lived, leading to the need to balance hydration with protein reinforcement by balancing the protein level. The **Protein Level™** in hair refers to the amount and quality of keratin and other structural proteins present in the cortex, the middle layer of the hair. Keratin, which makes up about 80% of the hair's structure, is a fibrous protein that provides strength, durability, and structural integrity. It acts as the hair's backbone, giving it the ability to withstand tension, maintain its shape, and resist breakage during styling or manipulation.

A healthy Protein Level ensures that the hair remains strong and resilient. It supports the hair's elasticity by providing a solid framework for the moisture to interact with, allowing the strands to stretch and return to their original form. When the Protein Level is compromised, hair becomes weak and fragile and more susceptible to damage, such as breakage, split ends, and excessive shedding.

Keratin treatments, deep conditioners, and leave-in conditioners are key to maintaining this Moisture and Protein balance. These products infuse the hair with moisture to enhance its ability to stretch and return to its original shape while also reinforcing the cortex with keratin or other proteins to provide structural integrity. A consistent routine that includes moisture-rich and protein-based treatments is critical to ensure the hair remains pliable, strong, and resilient. Additionally, the use of oils and emollients can help seal in moisture, preventing dehydration and protecting the hair from environmental stressors. These products create a barrier on the hair shaft, locking in hydration and preserving the flexibility of the strands. By balancing moisture with protein reinforcement and minimizing exposure to damaging practices, hair remains elastic, strong, and able to withstand everyday wear and tear, forming the foundation for healthy, manageable hair.

Hair Elasticity can be categorized into three levels: high elasticity, medium elasticity, and low elasticity, each reflecting the hair's ability to stretch and return to its original form without breaking. High elasticity indicates that the hair is in excellent health, with an optimal balance of moisture and protein. This hair type stretches significantly, often up to 50% of its length when wet, and quickly returns to its original shape. Hair with high elasticity is strong, resilient, and less prone to breakage, making it ideal for styles that require significant manipulation, such as braiding or curling.

Medium elasticity indicates that the hair is generally healthy but may show early signs of imbalance between moisture and protein. Hair with medium elasticity stretches under tension and returns close to its original shape, although not as effectively as hair with high elasticity. This condition often results from mild damage caused by heat styling, manipulation, or environmental stress. Fortunately, medium elasticity can usually be improved with regular deep conditioning treatments and occasional protein treatments to strengthen the hair structure. However, it's important to maintain balance; over-moisturizing can lead to hygral fatigue, a condition where the hair shaft becomes weakened from excessive swelling and contracting of the cuticle layers. Likewise, excessive protein use can lead to protein overload, making hair brittle, prone to breakage, and increased shedding. Careful observation and balanced care are key to restoring and maintaining optimal elasticity.

Low elasticity, on the other hand, is a sign of weakened or damaged hair. Hair in this category stretches very little, contracts very little, and often breaks when pulled. This can result from overprocessing with chemical treatments, excessive heat exposure, health issues, product buildup, protein overload, or prolonged dryness, which compromise the hair's cortex and cuticle layers. Low elasticity requires a targeted regimen that focuses on truly cleansing the surface of the hair, replenishing moisture to restore the hair's flexibility, and/ or repairing the cortex with protein-rich treatments. Understanding these levels of elasticity helps tailor a care routine to maintain or improve its Elasticity.

**How to Conduct a Hair Elasticity Test**

Testing hair's elasticity is an essential step to understanding its strength, flexibility, and overall health. Follow these simple steps to perform an elasticity test:

## ELASTICITY TEST

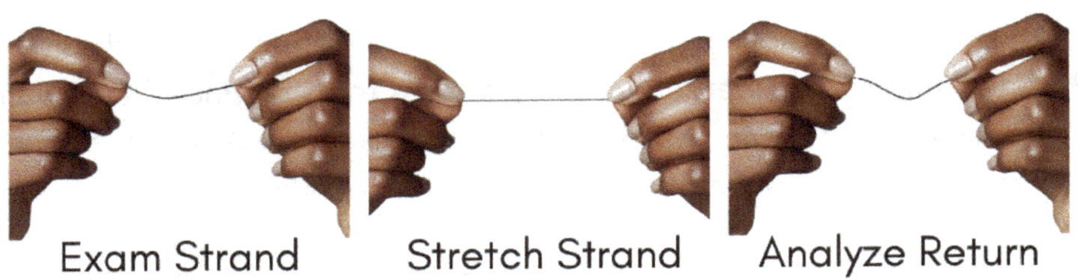


1. **Prepare the Hair:**
    - Ensure it is clean and free from product buildup, as this can affect the results.
    - Select strands from different areas of the head for a comprehensive assessment:
    - Organize each strand on a white piece of paper and write the area of the head from which each strand came.
2. **Examine the Strand:**
    - Select a strand, holding each end of the strand between your thumbs and pointer fingers without tension.
    - Observe the strand's initial length, shape, and thickness. Note any irregularities, such as thinning or uneven texture.
3. **Stretch the Strand:**
    - Slowly stretch the strand by pulling both ends in opposite directions. Be careful not to pull too quickly, as this may cause unnecessary breakage.
    - Observe how far the strand stretches without breaking.
4. **Analyze the Return:**
    - Release the strand and check if it returns to its original length, shape, and thickness.
        - If the strand stretches significantly and returns to its original state, the hair likely has high elasticity.

- If the strand somewhat gives and has a little stretch, but it maintains its original state, the hair likely has medium elasticity.
- If the strand stretches very little or breaks, the hair has low elasticity.

5. **Repeat the Test:**
   - Perform the test on strands from each section of your head to identify any variations in elasticity. Hair health can differ across the scalp, so this step is crucial for an accurate assessment.

This test allows you to analyze the hair's elasticity and adjust your hair care routine accordingly.

## Why Hair Elasticity Is An Important Property

Imagine your hair is like a rubber band. The rubber band needs flexibility (from moisture) and durability (from protein/strength) to function properly. If the rubber band becomes too wet or overly moisturized, it may stretch too far and lose its ability to snap back, becoming weak. On the other hand, if it becomes dry or brittle (lacking moisture) and loses its flexibility, it will pop under pressure. For the rubber band (or your hair) to work effectively, it needs the right balance of moisture to keep it pliable, while protein ensures it holds its shape and resists breakage.

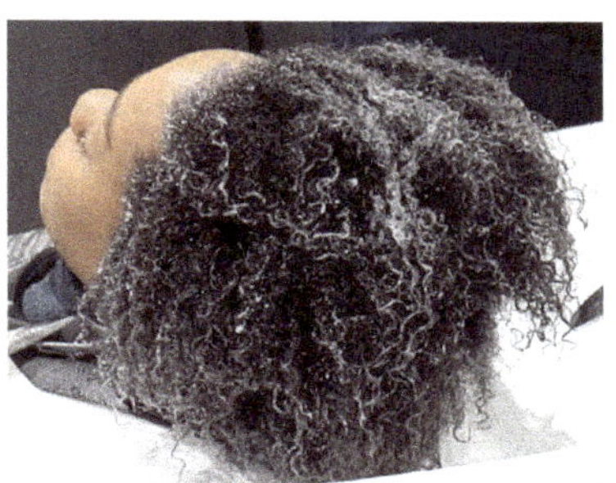

*Loss of Elasticity*

Knowing hair elasticity is crucial in caring for hair textures because highly textured hair can be extremely fragile due to the bends and turns exposed up and down the hair shaft. Hair elasticity determines how well it can stretch and recover during styling processes such as braiding, wash and gos, or heat styling. Hair with high elasticity can handle these manipulations with minimal risk of breakage, making it easier to achieve and maintain through thermal manipulation and protective styles. On the other hand, low-elasticity hair is more prone to snapping under tension, requiring extra care to avoid damage. By assessing elasticity, hair professionals can identify whether the hair needs more hydration, protein reinforcement, or both to improve its resilience, as well as communicate which styling options best serve the hair’s condition. Incorporating routine elasticity tests allows the professional to monitor the hair's health, make informed decisions about treatments, and maintain a regimen that promotes strength, flexibility, and long-term manageability.

### The Importance of Advancing Balanced Elasticity – Build, Balance, Maintain

ADVANCING BALANCED ELASTICITY
Build • Balance • Maintain
Balance Elasticity
Conduct Elasticity Test
Alternate Protein & Moisture Treatments
Build Elasticity
Reconstruct
Hydrate
Maintain Elasticity
Consistent Regimen, Reduce Mechanical Stress, Avoid Harmful Practices

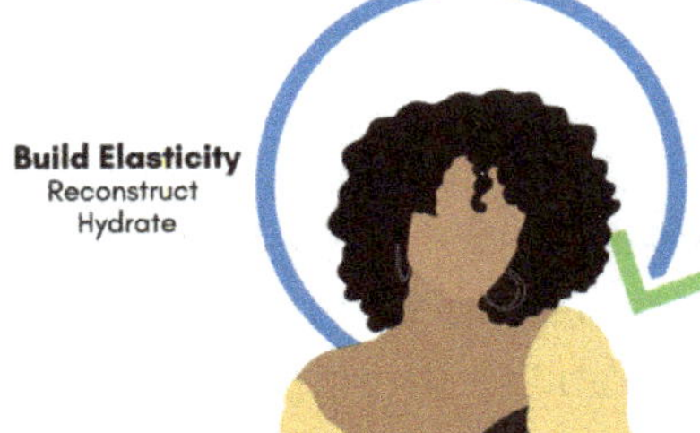

Establishing a healthy level of elasticity is not a one-time event but an ongoing commitment to maintaining optimal hair health. To ensure long-term resilience, strength, and manageability, professionals must consistently implement practices that build, balance, and maintain the hair's elastic potential. Building elasticity involves reconstructing the hair's internal structure with protein-rich treatments such as keratin masks, amino acid complexes, and hydrolyzed protein formulas. At the same time, it's essential to rehydrate dry strands with deep moisturizing treatments that infuse the hair with water and nutrients, and to use gentle detangling and low-tension techniques to minimize unnecessary breakage. Balancing elasticity requires alternating between protein and moisture-based products according to the hair's current condition, conducting regular elasticity tests to prevent protein overload or hygral fatigue, and adjusting treatments as needed to accommodate environmental influences like humidity, heat, or wind, as well as variations in styling practices. Maintaining elasticity involves establishing a consistent care regimen that includes weekly or biweekly conditioning, reducing mechanical stress while preserving hydration, and educating clients about harmful practices such as overuse of heat and chemical processing. When these steps are combined, hair becomes not only more elastic but also more resilient, manageable, and better prepared for styling challenges.

## Density

Hair **Density** refers to the number of hair strands per square inch of the scalp. It is the foundational factor in determining the fullness and overall appearance of hair, and the methods of styling used to ensure a balanced look.

- **High Density**: Indicates a high number of hair strands packed into a square inch of scalp. The hair appears full, thick, and voluminous. This type of density often supports more intricate hairstyles and creates a natural "bulk" even without styling.
- **Medium Density**: A standard number of hair strands per square inch of scalp. This results in a moderate amount of volume. Medium density allows for versatile styling but may require products or techniques to enhance fullness.
- **Low Density**: Refers to fewer hairs per square inch of scalp. This results in thinner-looking hair or areas where the scalp is more visible. Low density can be managed with lightweight products and techniques that create the illusion of volume.

The perception of hair density often differs with varying hair texture shapes (straight, wavy, curly, coily), influencing the perceived volume of hair. For instance, someone

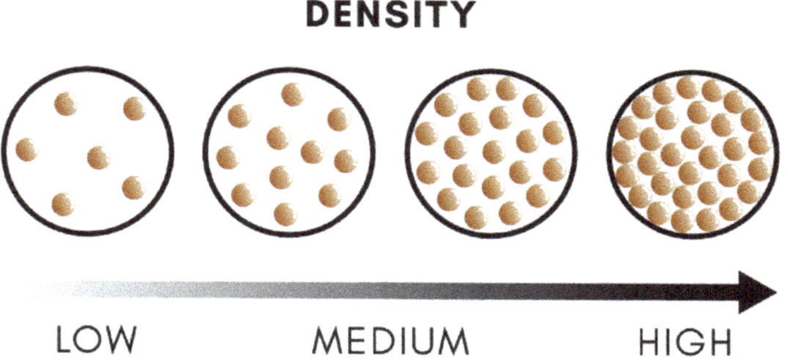


with fine hair may appear to have more volume when the hair is curly than when it is straightened. The density of highly textured hair is often best perceived when the hair is wet, rather than dry.

## Factors That Influence Hair Density

Hair density varies widely among individuals due to genetics, ethnicity, age, gender, diseases and disorders, hormonal changes, and the areas of the scalp.

### Genetics

Genetics is the primary factor determining how densely your hair grows. Each person is born with a specific number of hair-producing follicles, pre-determined by DNA. While lifestyle and hair care can influence the health of hair, they cannot increase the number of strands you are genetically predisposed to have. Genetics also determines the length of the hair's growth cycle as well as the speed of its growth rate. However, proper maintenance can help optimize the appearance of your natural density by reducing breakage and promoting healthy growth, and proper scalp treatments can revitalize dormant follicles to begin producing.

### Ethnicity

Different populations and ethnic groups tend to have genetic norms in variations of hair density:

- Caucasian hair typically has higher density.
- Asian hair often has slightly lower density but coarser strands.
- African hair tends to have the lowest density but more compact curls, creating an illusion of fullness.

### Age

As we age, hair density naturally declines due to changes in the hair growth cycle. The anagen (growth) phase of the hair cycle shortens over time, leading to less active hair growth. Additionally, the resting phase (telogen) becomes longer, which increases the likelihood of shedding without immediate replacement. These changes result in a gradual reduction in the number of visible hair strands on the scalp, creating the appearance of thinner hair. This is part of the natural aging process and affects most people to varying degrees. Aging also affects hair density indirectly through changes in overall health and scalp conditions. Reduced circulation to the scalp, declining collagen production, and nutritional deficiencies associated with aging can weaken hair strands and increase breakage, giving the impression of lower density.

**Diseases and Disorders**

Medical conditions like alopecia, thyroid dysfunction, high blood pressure, or stress-related hair loss can become prevalent causes of loss in density. Proper care by a medical professional, the use of nourishing hair products, maintaining a balanced diet, rest, and managing mental health can help prevent or reduce hair loss.

**Hormonal Changes**

Hormones regulate how long hair remains in the growth phase and influence whether hair follicles remain active or become dormant. Shifts in hormone levels due to life stages, medical conditions, or external factors can lead to noticeable changes in hair density. The four most common hormonal shifts that affect hair density include:

- **Puberty**: During puberty, increased levels of androgens, such as testosterone, can stimulate hair growth in some areas, such as facial or body hair, but may also lead to subtle thinning on the scalp in predisposed individuals.
- **Pregnancy and Postpartum**: High levels of estrogen during pregnancy prolong the growth phase, leading to thicker, fuller hair. After childbirth, estrogen levels drop and can advance the shedding phase, causing temporary thinning or postpartum hair loss.
- **Menopause**: During menopause, shifts in estrogen and progesterone levels often create hormonal imbalances that lead to hair thinning in women.
- **Hair Recession**: Also known as patterned hair loss, can often be linked to Dihydrotestosterone (DHT), a hormone that causes progressive shrinking of hair-producing follicles. This leads to shorter, finer hair strands and eventually stops hair growth entirely in affected areas.

## How to Determine Hair Density

To determine Density, you would assess the scalp and its distribution of follicles. To do this, create a clean part in your hair. It can be down the middle, to the side, or in any section that allows you to clearly see the scalp. Stand in good lighting and look directly at that part. If your density is low, the scalp line appears wide and open. The space between the strands is noticeable, and the scalp seems to dominate what you see. The hair appears to sit farther apart, almost as if each strand is standing on its own. In this case, you are seeing more scalp than hair along the part.

When your density is medium, the scalp is clearly visible, but it does not dominate. The part is present, defined, and easy to see, yet it does not appear wide or exaggerated. The strands sit close enough together to create fullness, but not so close that they conceal the scalp. There is a visual balance. The scalp and the hair share the space evenly.

If your density is high, the opposite happens. The scalp line becomes narrow, sometimes barely visible at all. The strands are closely packed together, crowding the part so tightly that the scalp is difficult to see. The hair takes up most of the visual space, leaving very little room for the scalp to show through. Here, you are seeing more hair than scalp.

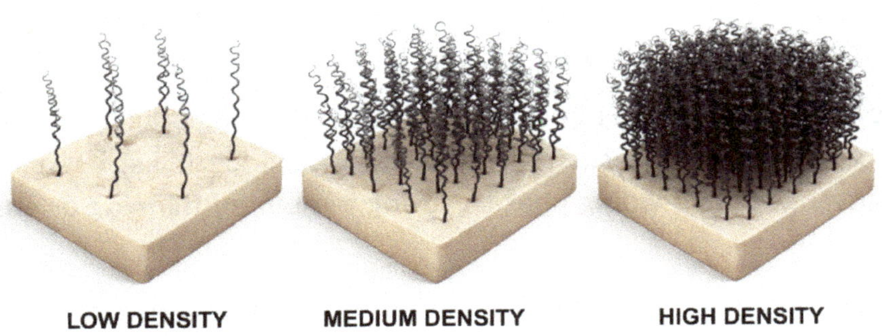


Hair density varies naturally across different areas of the scalp due to differences in follicular distribution. For instance, the occipital region (the back of the scalp) typically has the highest hair density, and the scalp perimeters have the lowest. Refer to the chapter on Scalp Spatial Distribution™ to learn how to map varying density by region.

## Porosity

Hair **Porosity** refers to the hair's ability to absorb, retain, and release moisture, determined by the placement and condition of the hair's cuticle. Hair porosity is the foundational trait that influences how your hair interacts with water and products, requiring a specific approach based on the Porosity Level. Similar to the scales of a pine cone, the cuticles of a hair strand open to varying degrees. The degree to which these cuticles open determines the hair porosity. Porosity levels are categorized as follows:

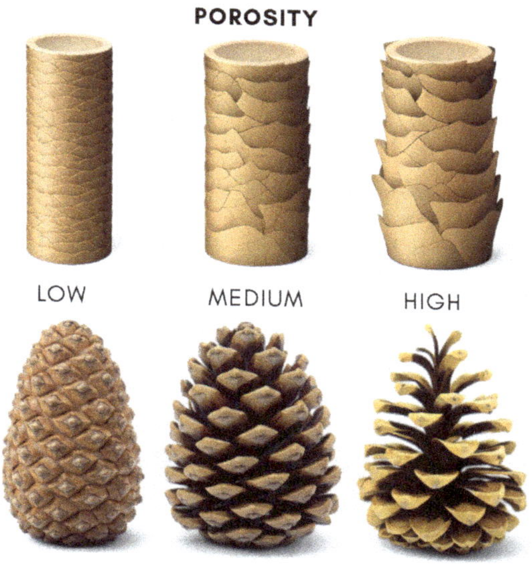

- **High Porosity**: Hair with the most open cuticle layer, highly raised or damaged, is often due to genetics, chemical treatments, or environmental stressors. This allows moisture to enter easily but escape just as quickly. Hair often feels dry, tangles easily, and is prone to frizz and breakage. High porosity hair requires special care to seal in moisture and prevent further damage.
- **Medium/Normal Porosity**: Hair with the normal placement of hair cuticles slightly raised is able to receive and release water and moisture. Hair with this porosity is generally healthy, shiny, and responsive to styling. Medium Porosity hair requires a balance of moisturizing and protein treatments as needed.
- **Low Porosity**: The cuticles are tightly packed and lie flat, making them resistant to accepting and releasing water. Water tends to bead up on the surface, and products may sit on the hair rather than absorb easily, leading to product buildup if not properly addressed. When styling Low Porosity hair, use lightweight, water-based products and apply moderate heat, when necessary, to open the cuticle for better absorption.

## Hair Porosity Analysis by Observation of Water Response

Observing how hair responds to water helps you evaluate its porosity. Oftentimes, hair responds to water differently in different areas. So, it's best to gather insight into absorption behavior across various areas of the scalp to gain a complete understanding of your overall texture profile. It is important to test on clarified hair for an accurate reading, as product buildup can skew the analysis.

1. On clarified dry hair, isolate a small section of hair
2. Lightly mist the strand with water
3. Observe how quickly the water is absorbed
4. Note whether water beads absorb slowly or absorb quickly
5. Repeat in another zone for comparison

Strands that absorb water quickly are considered High Porosity. Strands that require extended time, warmth, or the need to work the water into the hair for absorption would be considered Low Porosity. Hair that responds between the two would be considered Medium Porosity.

## Hair Porosity Analysis by Feel

While porosity is associated with how hair responds to water, the hair's feel can also provide valuable clues about the condition of the cuticle layer and its porosity level. By gently sliding your fingers along individual strands from the ends toward the scalp, you can observe whether the strand surface feels smooth, slightly textured, or noticeably rough.

A smoother feel may indicate a more aligned cuticle layer, indicating low porosity. A slightly textured feel may suggest moderate cuticle lifting, indicating medium porosity. A rough or uneven feel may indicate a more lifted cuticle layer, indicating high porosity.

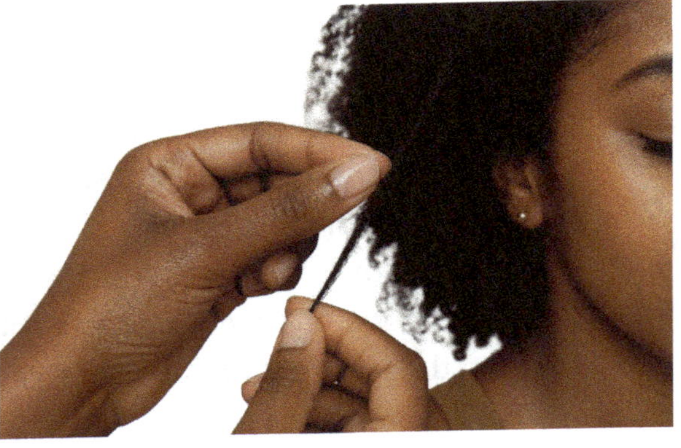

It is important to remember that feel-based observations do not independently determine porosity. Strand diameter, texture movement, chemical history, heat exposure, product residue, and environmental conditions can all influence how hair feels. For this reason, the most accurate assessment comes from combining feel-based observations with water-response observations and comparisons across multiple hair zones.

## A Commonly Used Conceptual Hair Porosity Test

The water test is a conceptual, yet effective way to determine your hair's porosity. By observing how your hair behaves in water, you can determine whether it has low, normal, or high porosity. Follow these steps:

### Materials Needed

- A clean, transparent glass or bowl
- Room-temperature water
- A few strands of clean, dry hair

### Steps By Step

1. **Start with Clean Hair:** Before performing the test, wash your hair with a clarifying shampoo to ensure it is free from product buildup, oils, and conditioners. Buildup can affect the accuracy of the test.
2. **Fill the Glass:** Fill the glass or bowl with room-temperature water. Avoid using hot or cold water, as this can affect the test results.
3. **Select Hair Strands:** Use a few strands of your hair. These can be strands naturally shed during combing or brushing. Hair from different parts of your head may have varying porosities, so consider testing and tracking the multiple strands.
4. **Drop the Hair in the Water:** Track each strand of hair and gently place it on the surface of the water. Avoid pushing them down, as this might skew the results.
5. **Observe for 2-4 Minutes:** Watch the hair to see how it reacts to the water. The behavior of the strands will indicate your hair porosity.

### Results

- **Low Porosity:** Hair floats on the surface and takes a long time to sink, if at all. This indicates tightly closed cuticles that resist water absorption.
- **Normal/Medium Porosity:** Hair slowly sinks to the middle of the glass. This indicates cuticles that absorb and retain moisture well, balancing hydration.

- **High Porosity:** Hair sinks quickly to the bottom of the glass. This indicates highly raised or damaged cuticles that easily absorb but struggle to retain moisture.

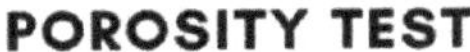


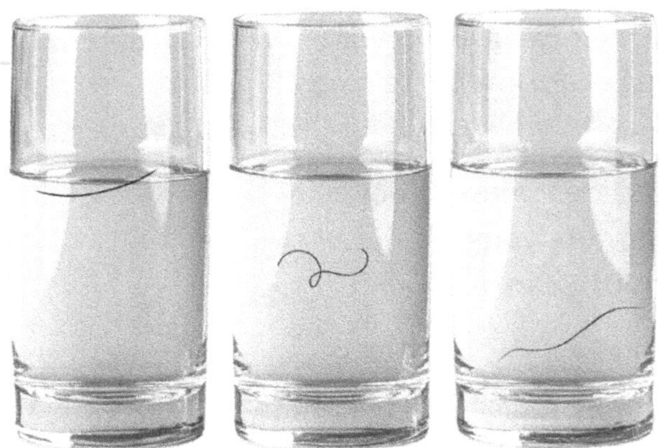

This test provides an indication of porosity, but it's helpful to combine it with how your hair feels and reacts to moisture in your daily routine to fully determine hair porosity.

**Caring for High Porosity Hair**

High porosity hair is vulnerable due to its raised or damaged cuticle structure. Without proper care, it can become brittle, leading to split ends, breakage, and further porosity issues. Gentle care and a strategic approach to moisture retention and strengthening are crucial for maintaining its health and promoting length retention. Here are some key tips:

- **Layering Products**: Apply products that first hydrate and then seal in the moisture. Start with water or a water-based leave-in, and then seal with an oil or an emollient to close the moisture beneath the cuticle. This is similar to, but not the same as, the LOC method developed by Rochelle Graham-Campbell, the founder and CEO of Alikay Naturals.

- **Protein Treatments**: Incorporate protein-rich products to temporarily fill in fractured cuticles or gaps between cuticles. This helps to protect the hair from excessive dehydration.

- **Sealing Cuticles**: To flatten the cuticle and retain moisture, finish with cool water rinses or acidic pH-balanced products (e.g., aloe vera juice or apple cider vinegar rinses), or a product containing porosity fillers.
- **Gentle Handling**: High porosity hair is more prone to breakage, so avoid excessive manipulation and tension.
- **Deep Conditioning**: Regularly deep condition with moisturizing and repairing treatments to improve elasticity and prevent dryness.
- **Protect from Heat and Environmental Damage**: When exposed to heat and harsh conditions, use heat protectants and cover hair with satin or silk.

**Caring for Medium Porosity Hair**

Medium porosity hair thrives on balance. It adapts well to treatments but requires proactive maintenance. Alternate moisture and strengthening masks as needed, and monitor hair behavior routinely. Avoid overloading with protein or oil

**Caring for Low Porosity Hair**

Low porosity hair presents three main challenges that may make maintenance tricky, including: moisture retention, protein overload, and product buildup. The challenge of moisture penetration, as the hair naturally resists water absorption, can lead to dryness and a lack of elasticity if not properly managed. To maintain healthy, hydrated hair, a tailored approach is necessary. Examples include:

- **Steaming**: Use a hair steamer during deep conditioning to lift the cuticle and encourage moisture absorption.
- **Warm Water Rinse**: Start your wash routine with warm water to lift the cuticle.
- **Clarify Regularly:** Use a gentle clarifying shampoo to remove product buildup that can block moisture penetration.
- **Humectants**: Use humectants like glycerin and aloe vera to attract and hold moisture.
- **Avoid Heavy Products**: Skip heavy butters, creams, and oils, which can sit on the surface of the hair.

The second challenge is protein sensitivity, as low porosity hair does not require excessive strengthening. Too much protein can cause the hair to become stiff, brittle, and prone to breakage. Understanding these challenges is key to developing a hair care routine that ensures proper hydration, lightweight product application, and balanced protein use to maintain healthy, vibrant hair.

Lastly, product buildup is a common issue, as it is an external layer of residue (from oils, butters, silicones, or other products) that physically blocks moisture from entering the hair shaft. This also causes heavy products to sit on the hair rather than penetrate the strands. This buildup can clog the cuticles, leaving the hair looking dull and weighed down. Select a lightweight, water-based products that won't leave a heavy residue on the hair or dilute heavy products that can sit on the surface of the hair. Look for leave-in conditioners, styling creams, or gels specifically formulated for low porosity hair. These products are designed to provide moisture without causing buildup. Also, use a gentle clarifying shampoo to remove product buildup that can block moisture penetration. This helps to maintain a healthy balance and ensures that your hair can receive the benefits of your chosen products without being hindered by buildup.

**Common Confusion Between Low Porosity and Product Buildup**

A delayed reaction to water, slow absorption, and slow saturation are indicators of low porosity. Product buildup often mimics low-porosity hair in the same way, leading to confusion about hair's actual porosity. Both scenarios result in products sitting on the hair surface, causing frustration and poor hair care results. This is why it is necessary to remove buildup from the hair when attempting to analyze porosity. Product buildup can easily be remedied by regular double cleansing, with a routine clarifying shampoo designed to remove buildup. Apple cider vinegar rinses can also be effective for gentle yet thorough cleansing. Frequency depends on how much of the product is routinely used. Heavy use of products like butters, oils, and gels can be clarified every 2 weeks, while light product usage can be clarified once a month.

By understanding and addressing hair porosity, you can develop a tailored routine that ensures hair thrives, staying moisturized, strong, and beautiful.

# Length

Hair **Length** is the measurement of hair from root to end. As a professional, it's essential to be able to communicate the ways hair length is categorized, from the perspective of its natural texture and behavior. These categories include True Length, Perceived Length, and the degree of Shrinkage. These categorizations help to manage expectations and account for the unique characteristics of hair textures, particularly shrinkage.

## Determining Hair Length

**True Length™** reflects the actual full length of hair strands when completely extended or straightened, whether by natural fall or techniques such as thermal straightening, blow-drying, banding, or pulling to stretch to the full length. **Perceived Length™** refers to how long the hair appears when it rests in its natural texture shape. This length is visible when highly textured hair is dry and settles without being stretched or straightened. Hair **Shrinkage** is the natural phenomenon in which hair contracts and appears shorter than its true length when fully stretched or straightened. This occurs because highly textured hair tends to contract and "shrink" into compact shapes. The **Degree of Shrinkage™** is the difference between the hair's True Length and its Perceived Length when the hair contracts to its natural texture shape. It is best to communicate both the perceived and stretched lengths when consulting with a highly textured hair client about haircuts and styling. Clarifying which length the client is referring to throughout a consultation ensures that the degree of shrinkage is taken into consideration.

There are 3 Degrees of Shrinkage:

- **High Degree of Shrinkage**: 90%-50% Length Contraction
- **Medium Degree of Shrinkage**: 50%-30% Length Contraction
- **Low Degree of Shrinkage**: 5%-30%  Length Contraction.

The Degree of Shrinkage can vary significantly, from person to person, based on each individual's Texture Shape. For example, wavy and loosely curly hair have a Low

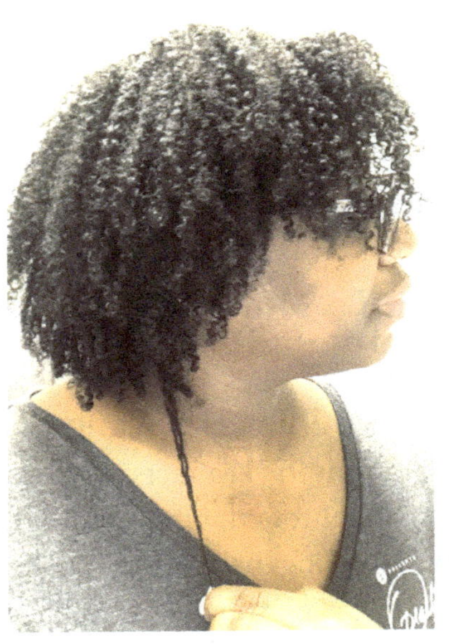

Degree of Shrinkage, retaining a larger proportion of their length. Curly and Looser Curly hair has a Medium Degree of Shrinkage, while tighter curls, coils, and kinks have a High Degree of Shrinkage and can shrink by as much as 50-90%, making the hair appear extremely shorter than it actually is. There are many people with kinky and coily texture shapes that have such a high Degree of shrinkage that their Perceived Length will always appear the same, regardless of how long their True Length grows. This is the key reason why it is vitally important for clients who desire a curly cut to arrive at their appointment with their hair dried and styled in their defined curl. This allows the stylist to assess the degree of shrinkage the client has and, therefore, determine the appropriate length of the cut and shape.

Shrinkage is a sign of healthy hair elasticity, as it reflects the hair's ability to revert to its natural texture shape after being manipulated. While some see shrinkage as a challenge because it hides the True Length of the hair, others embrace it as a unique trait of highly textured hair that contributes to its volume and versatility.

## DEGREES OF SHRINKAGE

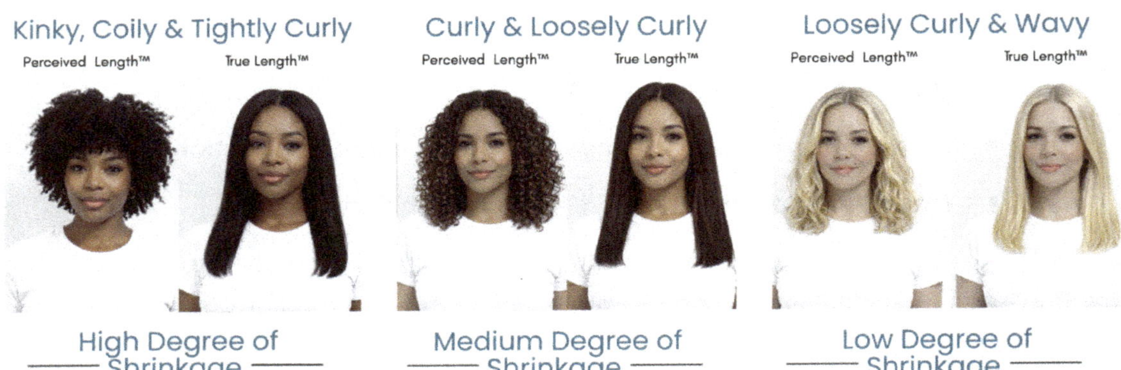

**Length Distinctions**

Referring to hair Length as long, short, or medium can be highly subjective, based on the communicator's perspective, culture, and experience with hair texture. For instance, someone with loosely curly or straight hair might perceive shoulder-length hair as short, whereas someone with kinky coily hair may view shoulder-length hair as long.

Understanding common length distinctions helps to standardize communication and manage expectations during consultations. Common length distinctions include:

**Short Hair**

- Close Cut: Hair length is a few millimeters long, also known as a Clipper Cut, Close-cropped, Buzz Cut, or Palm Roll length.
- Ear Length: Hair extends just to the bottom of the earlobe.
- Chin Length: Hair reaches the chin, framing the face.

**Mid-Length Hair**

- Neck Length: Hair falls to around the base of the neck or collarbone.
- Shoulder Length: Hair grazes or rests on or just below the ridge of the shoulders.

**Long Hair**

- Mid Back Length: Hair falls beyond the shoulders to the middle of the back, around the bra strap.
- Waist Length: Hair reaches the natural waistline.
- Beyond Waist Length: Hair extends past the waist, including hip, thigh, or even floor-length styles.

# HAIR LENGTHS

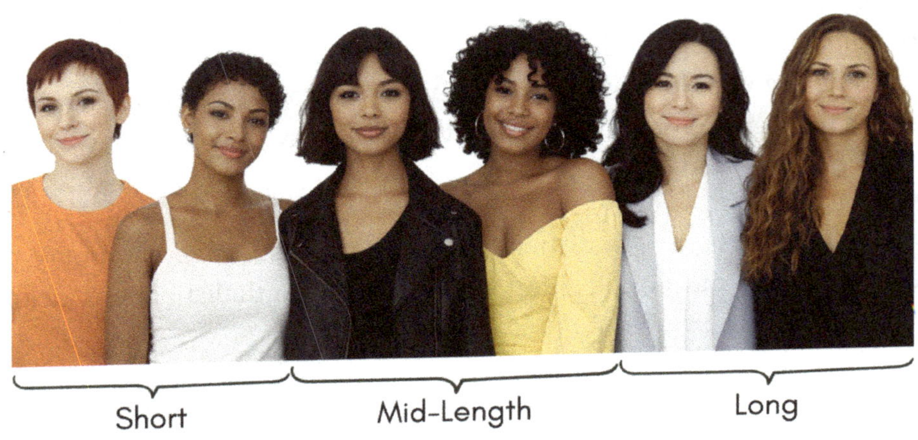


**Identifying Hair Growth Rate & Projecting Length Retention**

Hair growth is a fundamental, yet often misunderstood, aspect of achieving and maintaining hair length, particularly within the highly textured hair community. Due to the natural shrinkage of curly and coily hair, many individuals become discouraged when they only see the Perceived Length that may reflect minimal growth. However, it's important to understand that hair is continuously growing. The focus shouldn't solely be on whether the hair is growing, but also on how well the hair that grows is retained.

Achieving hair length goals depends on two interconnected factors: a healthy growth rate and effective length retention. Growth refers to the biological process occurring at the scalp, while retention focuses on preserving the ends of the hair, the oldest and most fragile part of the strand. Without proper retention practices, even healthy growth can appear stagnant. In this way, growth and retention are truly two sides of the same coin, both essential for realizing long, healthy hair.

**Growth Rate**

Hair growth occurs in three distinct phases: **Anagen** (the active growth phase), **Catagen** (the transitional phase), and **Telogen** (the resting phase). **Growth Rate™** refers to the rate at which an individual's hair grows and is influenced by several factors, including genetics, hormonal activity, age, overall health, and, in some cases, medication. Under normal, healthy conditions, the average human grows approximately ¼ to ½ inches of hair each month or 3 to 6 inches annually. However, this is a general standard, not a universal measurement. Some individuals may consistently grow nearer to ½ inches per month, while others may average ¼ inches or less. Both rates fall within the normal range for hair growth.

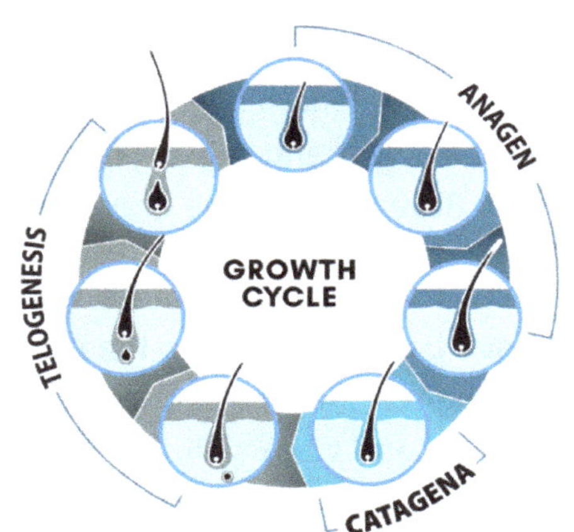


As a professional, it is vitally important to understand that hair growth is highly individualized and that genetic predisposition significantly influences variations among your clients. Establishing a client's baseline growth rate through observation and consistent measurement over time facilitates realistic goal-setting and accurate progress assessments. One effective method for determining a client's baseline growth rate is to take monthly measurements of a specific, stretched section of hair, preferably from the nape. Using tools such as length-check T-shirts, growth charts, or standardized photo documentation captured monthly can help track progress and account for the effects of shrinkage, especially in tight textured hair types, where coils, curls, and waves may obscure visible length. Emphasizing stretch-based measurement rather than relying solely on observations ensures a more accurate understanding of true hair growth and supports healthy expectations for both clients and stylists. Once you have identified the Growth Rate, you can begin to make realistic length projections. For instance, let's use the standard growth rate of about ½ inch per month; you can expect approximately 1.5 inches of growth in three months, 3 inches in six months, and 6 inches in a year. Making these projections is not an exact science;

rather, it serves as a gauge with a high degree of subjectivity. These projections can be made assuming minimal breakage and consistent care.

## Length Retention

The second key factor in meeting length goals is **Length Retention**, the ability to preserve hair length by preventing breakage, damage, and splitting at the ends of the hair, the oldest and most fragile part of the strand. Without intentional practices for Length Retention, all the growth in the world won't translate to visible length.

Regular trims are crucial in ensuring Length Retention. Hair constantly experiences damage from exposure to the elements, friction, heat exposure, dryness, and regular wear and tear. All of this causes fractures on the hair shaft and ends, resulting in splits, breakage, and weak points. By proactively trimming away these worn ends every 90 days or once a season, you prevent damage from setting in and expanding up the hair shaft. This aids in ensuring that trims require the least amount of hair as possible. Going an extended period of time without trimming the ends may cause unnecessary damage, resulting in more hair needing to be cut and the appearance of little to no hair growth. Trims should strategically be done to avoid and remove split ends, single-strand knots, and irreparable frayed ends, similar to pruning a cared-for plant, allowing it to thrive. However, excessive trimming should be avoided. Signs that indicate that hair needs trimming include:

- Thinning Ends
- Split Ends
- Dry and Frizzy Ends
- Single-Strand Knots
- Ends that refuse to curl or hold in styles
- Ends that are a looser texture than the hair, mid to root of the hair shaft

There are three standard types of trims commonly used in highly textured hair care: Shaping, Healthy Trimming, and Dusting.

- Shaping is typically performed on wet or dry hair when the ends are relatively healthy. This type of trim is intended to maintain the desired shape or silhouette of the style, focusing on refining the perimeter of the hair without extensive interior cutting. It is often considered a basic haircut and is usually priced accordingly by stylists.

- Healthy Trimming is a more corrective approach, done on either wet or blown-out hair. The primary purpose of this trim is to remove all damaged, split, or compromised ends, regardless of the amount of hair that needs to be cut. This type of trimming prioritizes the health and longevity of the hair over length retention and may result in a more noticeable reduction in length.
- Dusting involves removing a minimal amount of hair, typically just the very tips. When performed on already healthy hair, dusting serves as a maintenance technique to prevent future damage and density. However, many clients request dusting as a substitute for a proper trim-out of fear that trimming will hinder their length goals. In these cases, not enough hair is removed to correct existing damage. This often leads to thin, weakened ends that tangle easily, split further, and become increasingly difficult to detangle or style. Ultimately, this can result in the need for a more substantial cut to restore hair health. To prevent this cycle, it's essential to educate clients on the purpose and timing of trims, helping them understand that strategic trimming supports, rather than sabotages, long-term hair growth and retention. Avoidance eventually leads to counterproductive results in the long run.

To determine how often you should trim ends, purposely monitor how long it takes for your hair to get excessively tangled, have single-strand knots, be frizzy, dry, or experience thinning ends. By determining the client's hair's pattern of wear and tear, you will get a general idea of how often their lifestyle requires the hair to be trimmed. Use this as a guide to proactively set a strategic routine of trimming before damage sets in.

**Hair Treatments For Healthy Hair Growth & Length Retention**

Hair treatments also play a major role in Length Retention. Hydration treatments keep curls pliable and reduce breakage. Protein treatments strengthen the hair shaft and help maintain structure. Lipids and occlusives replenish and seal in hair's moisture.

Keep in mind that scalp care significantly influences hair growth by fostering a healthy environment for hair follicles to function optimally. When the scalp is clean, balanced, and well-nourished, blood circulation improves, inflammation decreases, and hair follicles are more likely to remain in the anagen phase longer, which promotes consistent, healthy hair growth. Key practices for maintaining a healthy scalp include regular cleanses, gentle exfoliation, gentle massages to promote blood flow to follicles, moisturization, antimicrobials, antifungal, and antioxidant ingredients, as well as maintaining the scalp's pH balance between 4.5 and 5.5.

Daily habits are as important as a consistent treatment plan. When done properly, protective styles can significantly enhance the ideal conditions for length retention and healthy hair growth. Low-manipulation styles, regular moisturizing and sealing, and sleeping on satin or silk can have a notable impact. Gentle detangling with the appropriate tools and minimizing excessive heat exposure can also promote length retention and healthy hair growth. Remember, what happens internally is just as crucial as what occurs externally, so maintaining a nutrient-rich diet, proper hydration, and effective stress management all contribute to healthy hair growth from the root up. By understanding how hair grows and what it needs to thrive, you'll be able to project not only growth potential but also the ability to retain every inch grown.

## Strand Diameter

**Strand Diameter™** refers to the width of an individual strand of hair and is categorized as fine, medium, or thick (coarse). The diameter affects hair's overall appearance, strength, and how it behaves during styling and care. Categories of Strand Diameter include:

- **Fine Hair**: Consists of thin, delicate strands that are often lightweight and prone to breakage. Fine hair has fewer layers of the cuticle and may not have a medulla layer to its structure, which makes it less resilient. This trait is prone to breakage and split ends, making length retention more challenging without gentle handling and protection. Looser texture, shaped hair can become oily quickly as sebum spreads easily, and it's more difficult to achieve voluminous styles due to its low density. This trait also holds styles like curls less effectively, often requiring lightweight products to avoid weighing it down.
- **Medium Hair**: The most common strand diameter is stronger and more versatile than fine hair, with an average number of cuticle layers. Medium Hair

generally has good length retention if properly cared for and is balanced, manageable, and less prone to damage. This trait can handle a variety of products, works well with most styles, and holds curls or straightening better than fine hair.

- **Thick (Coarse) Hair:** Consists of large-diameter strands that are strong and resistant to breakage. Has the highest number of cuticle layers. Coarse hair retains length easily due to its strength, but can be prone to dryness, which can lead to breakage if not moisturized adequately. This trait is more resistant to chemical treatments and takes longer to dry or style. This trait holds styles well and often requires heat or stronger hold products to achieve sleek looks.

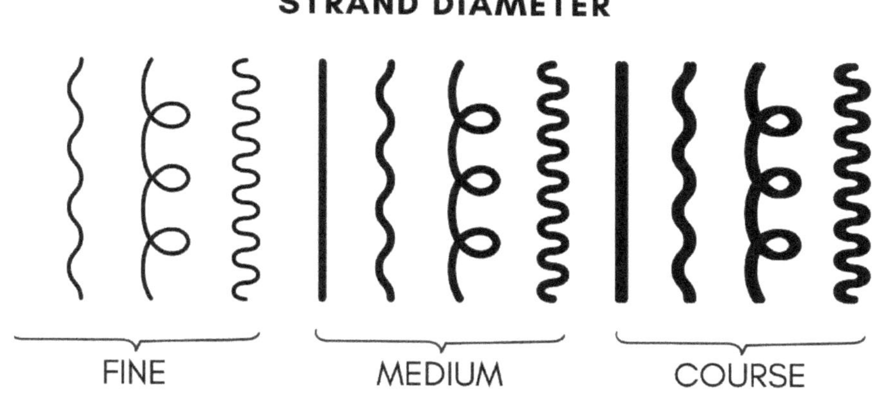


These categories range greatly. An adult hair strand is approximately 20–180 µm (0.02–0.18 mm) wide. In comparison, an average cotton sewing thread is 100–200 µm (0.10–0.20 mm).

**How To Identify Your Strand Diameter**

To identify your Strand Diameter, take a strand of hair between your thumb and your index finger. Slide your fingers down the hair strand. If you can distinctly feel the strand, your strand is coarse or thick. If it's hard to feel the strands between your fingers, your strands are fine.

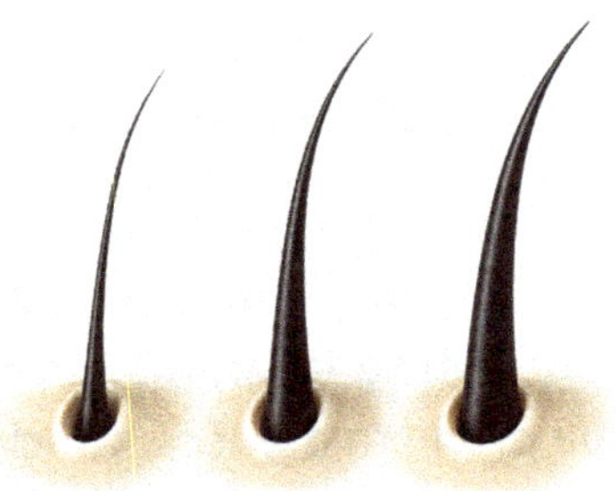

You can also compare how your Strand Diameter varies in the various zones of your head. To compare, select a strand from varying zones of the scalp and lay it on a white sheet of paper. Compare the thickness of each strand to the other. These determinations will help you understand how much your hair can handle, how much product to use, and even which products to use.

**How Strand Diameter Affects Different Texture Shapes**

Strand Diameter greatly affects both the lived-in experience and the aesthetics of different texture shapes. These factors influence everything from styling longevity to volume, curl definition, how hair reacts to products, humidity, and environmental conditions. You may find that Fine strands struggle with holding styles and can be easily overwhelmed by heavy products. Medium strands offer the best balance between volume, definition, and ease of care. Thick strands maintain shape and structure well but require more time to dry, style, and absorb moisture effectively. Here are some key effects that Strand Diameter has on varying Texture Shapes:

**Straight Hair & Strand Diameter**

- **Fine:** It lies flat and lacks volume, often becoming oily quickly. Due to low structural support, styles may fall flat easily.
- **Medium:** Holds shape better, offering a smoother yet fuller appearance. More resistant to oiliness than fine strands.
- **Thick:** Can appear heavy and resistant to styling (e.g., curling). It has a more naturally sleek, glass-like finish, but may take longer to dry.

**Wavy Hair & Strand Diameter**

- **Fine:** Forms soft, barely-there waves that can lose definition quickly, especially in humidity. It can easily be weighed down by heavy products.
- **Medium:** More defined waves with a balance between volume and movement. Holds styles moderately well.
- **Thick:** Has bold, structured waves but can be heavy, causing waves to stretch or loosen. More resistant to frizz, but can feel bulky.

**Curly Hair & Strand Diameter**

- **Fine:** Forms soft, airy curls that are prone to frizz and loss of definition. Needs a lightweight but strong hold to maintain shape.
- **Medium:** Holds curls well with a balance of bounce and volume. Manages frizz moderately.
- **Thick:** Forms bold, well-structured curls that retain their shape longer.

**Coily/Kinky Hair & Strand Diameter**

- **Fine:** Forms delicate, tight coils or zigzags that shrink significantly and are highly prone to breakage and dehydration. Requires gentle handling and layering of hydration.
- **Medium:** Holds shape well while maintaining a balance of volume and elasticity. It's more resilient but still needs significant moisture.
- **Thick:** Creates dense, structured coils that have excellent volume but can be more challenging to fully hydrate and detangle. Requires products with a stronger hold.

**Incongruent Textures & Strand Diameter**

- **Fine:** The differences in texture are more apparent. Some sections may not hold styles as well as other sections.
- **Medium:** Texture inconsistencies blend more naturally, allowing for even styling and better shape retention.
- **Thick:** May have a strong contrast between different textures. It can be more challenging to shape uniformly, but it offers visual depth that is aesthetically pleasing.

**How Strand Diameter Influences Other Hair Properties**

There are no distinct rules on how Strand Diameter works interchangeably with other hair traits. However, there are some commonalities that you may observe, which often reflect how Strand Diameter may influence other properties and affect the lived-in experience and overall aesthetics of the hair.

- **Porosity & Strand Diameter**

  Fine strands typically have a higher porosity, as their cuticle layers are thinner and more prone to moisture loss, making them susceptible to dryness and frizz.

Medium strands have moderate porosity, retaining moisture more efficiently while balancing hydration and absorption. Thick strands, with their stronger cuticle structure, often have lower porosity, making it harder for moisture to penetrate but also preventing rapid moisture loss, which can result in longer-lasting hydration.

- **Density & Strand Diameter**
  Fine strands, even in high-density hair, can appear flat or less voluminous, requiring volumizing products to enhance fullness. Medium strands provide a balanced density, offering a naturally full look without excessive bulk. Thick strands create naturally high-density aesthetics, often appearing full and voluminous even with fewer strands per square inch, though they may feel heavier and require more effort to manage.

- **Elasticity & Strand Diameter**
  Fine strands tend to have lower elasticity, meaning they can snap easily when stretched, making them more prone to breakage and requiring extra strengthening treatments. Medium strands have moderate elasticity, allowing for a good balance of stretch and resilience, making them easier to style and manipulate. Thick strands have higher elasticity, meaning they can stretch significantly without breaking, making them more resistant to damage but sometimes more challenging to style due to their structural resistance.

- **Shrinkage & Strand Diameter**
  Shrinkage is most prominent in curly and coily hair, where strand diameter affects how tightly the hair coils. Fine strands commonly experience higher shrinkage, as their delicate nature allows coils to contract more. Medium strands commonly shrink at a moderate rate, maintaining shape while retaining some length. Thick strands often resist shrinkage, as their weight naturally elongates the texture shape, giving the appearance of longer hair even in its natural state.

**Product Knowledge For Varying Strand Diameters**

For straight hair, fine strands tend to get oily quickly and struggle with volume, requiring volumizing sulfate-free shampoos, lightweight conditioners with protein, and root-lifting mousses. Medium strands benefit from balancing shampoos, lightweight hydration with panthenol or aloe vera, and light serums for smoothness. Thick strands often appear sleek but can be heavy and resistant to styling, making strong to medium-hold styling products essential.

Wavy hair requires hydration without excessive weight. Fine wavy strands need gentle shampoos, lightweight protein-infused conditioners, and salt sprays or mousses for soft definition. Medium strands hold waves better with moisturizing shampoos, curl creams, and medium-hold gels to enhance movement. Thick, wavy strands, which can stretch under their own weight, benefit from deep hydration, moderate oils, and oil-based conditioners, and humidity-resistant serums to maintain structure.

For curly hair, maintaining a balance of moisture and definition is key. Fine curly strands are prone to frizz and losing curl definition easily. They do well with lightweight, moisture-rich shampoos, foams, and flexible-hold gels. Medium strands retain curls better and respond well to hydrating shampoos, humectant-rich leave-in conditioners, and curl-defining creams and gels. Thick curly strands form bold, structured curls that require deep moisture shampoos, oils, curl butters, and strong-hold gels for definition and longevity.

Coily and kinky hair experiences dryness and requires intense hydration and elasticity support. Fine, coily strands thrive with sulfate-free shampoos, protein-balanced conditioners, and lightweight creams or mousse-based stylers. Medium strands need deep conditioning with penetrating oils like coconut or castor oil paired with butter-based creams and medium-hold gels. Thick strands benefit from co-washing or sulfate-free shampoos, heavy deep conditioning treatments, rich butters, and protective styling serums to maintain moisture and elasticity.

For incongruent texture, where inconsistent patterns coexist, customized care is essential. Fine strands benefit from hydrating yet lightweight shampoos, soft-hold gels, and leave-in mists to unify textures. Medium strands require balanced hydration with flexible conditioning, medium-hold curl creams, and styling foams. Thick strands need intense hydration from heavy conditioners and oils, layered with strong-hold gels and sealing oils to maintain consistency across different curl or wave patterns. It is all about finding a happy medium.

In general, Fine strands require lightweight hydration and flexible hold products to avoid being weighed down. Medium strands thrive with balanced moisture and structured stylers. Thick strands demand deep hydration and strong-hold stylers for long-lasting manageability. Understanding these nuances helps in selecting the best products to enhance the natural beauty and health of each hair type.

## Key Terms

**Hair Properties:** Specific hair traits that determine hair's appearance, behavior, and overall health, including Elasticity, Density, Porosity, and Length.

**Elasticity**: The hair's ability to stretch and return to its original shape without breaking.

**Moisture Level™:** The amount of water content within the hair strands.

**Protein Level™:** The amount and quality of keratin and other structural proteins present in the cortex, the middle layer of the hair

**Density**: The number of hair strands per square inch of the scalp.

**Porosity:** The hair's ability to absorb, retain, and release moisture.

**Length**: The measurement of hair from root to end.

**True Length™**: The actual full length of hair strands when completely extended or straightened.

**Perceived Length™:** The amount and quality of keratin and other structural proteins present in the cortex.

**Shrinkage™**: The natural phenomenon in which textured hair contracts and appears shorter than its true length when fully stretched or straightened.

**Degree of Shrinkage™**: The difference between the hair's True Length and its Perceived Length when the hair contracts to its natural texture shape.

**Anagen**: The active phase of the Growth Cycle.

**Catagen**: The resting phase of the Growth Cycle.

**Telogen**: The resting phase of the Growth Cycle.

**Growth Rate™**: The rate at which an individual's hair grows.

**Length Retention™**: The ability to preserve hair length.

**Strand Diameter™**: The width of an individual strand of hair.

# Texture Dynamics - Pillar 2

# TEXTURE INDICATORS™

## HAIR PRESENTATION

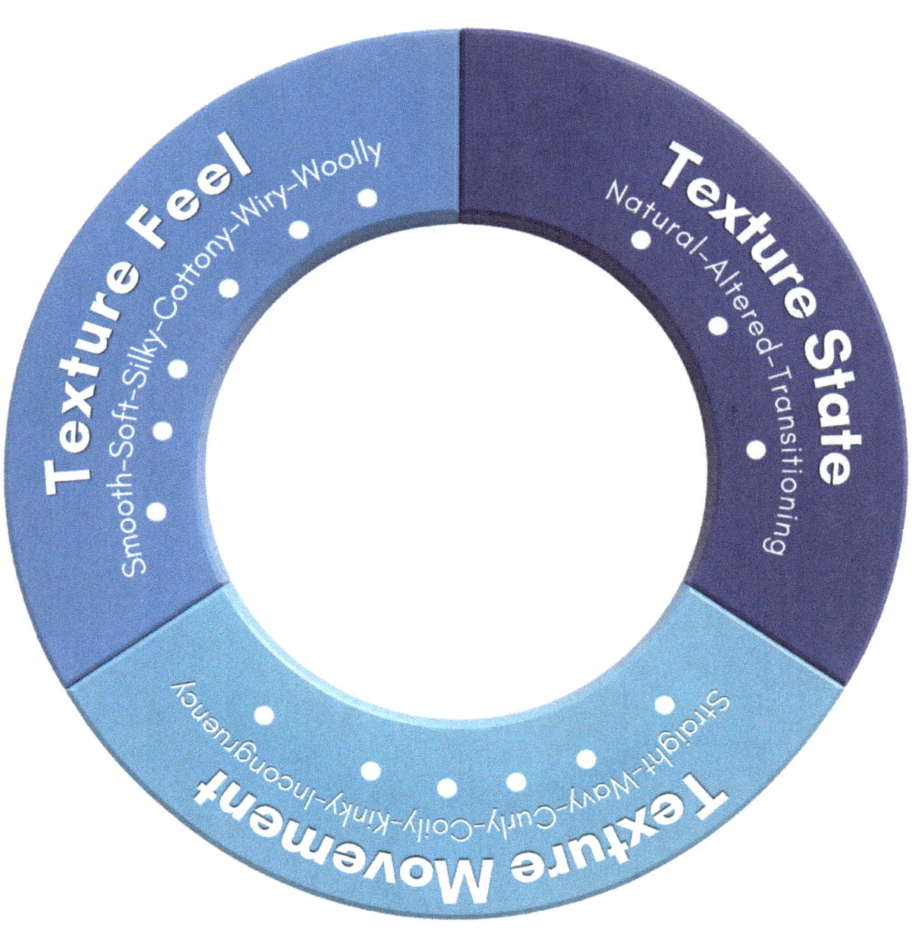

# 4.
# Pillar 2 - Texture Indicators™

*How various hair characteristics interact and work together to influence the Hair Texture.*

To effectively understand Texture Dynamics, we must first definitively understand how the term Hair Texture is used in real-life applications. In salon and layman's terms, Hair Texture refers to the overall appearance and tactile experience of the hair, interchangeably describing the shape, movement, and feel. **Texture Indicators™** are the various hair characteristics that interact and work together to influence the Hair Texture, its overall appearance, behavior, styling options, and hair care needs. These characteristics consist of:

- **Texture State™:** The distinction between natural, altered, and transitioning hair.
- **Texture Movement™:** The shape and pattern of hair curvature and bend.
- **Texture Feel™:** Characteristics of hair that can be observed by touch.

Texture Dynamics™ are in constant flux due to internal and external factors, showing that no two heads of hair are exactly alike. By gaining a comprehensive understanding of each client's Texture Dynamics, hair professionals can tailor hair care routines and maximize their clients' styling potential.

## Texture State™

When disulfide bonds in the hair are permanently broken, the hair's structure changes, resulting in a shift from its natural state to an altered one. This change in the hair's state causes the hair to no longer behave the way it did naturally. **Texture State** refers to the current state of an individual's hair in comparison to its original natural structure, classified into three categories: Natural, Altered, or Transitioning. **Natural Hair**, also known as virgin hair, is hair that retains its original structure and characteristics. It is unaltered and free from substantial interventions like permanent chemical processes, thermal treatments, or significant damage that alter its natural structure, including texture shape, and texture pattern. Conversely, **Altered Hair™** has undergone a permanent change to its natural structure due to factors such as high-heat styling, chemical treatments (including relaxers, perms, or color processes), excessive tension, or manipulation, resulting in extensive damage or a fundamentally different texture compared to its original form.

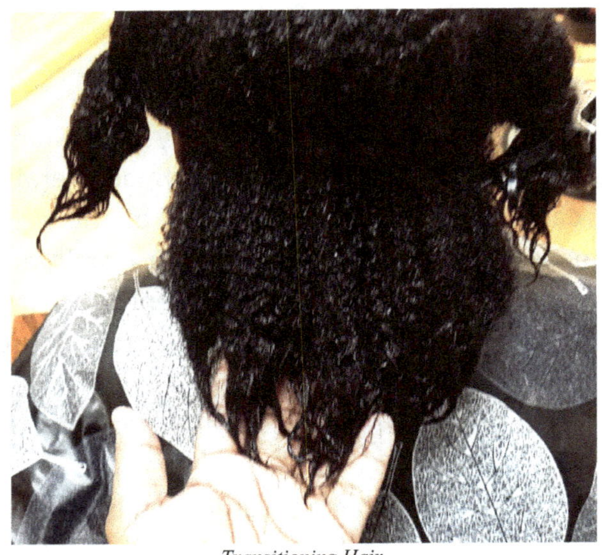
*Transitioning Hair*

**Transitioning Hair** in a mixed state, where natural texture is growing in at the roots, but altered hair remains on the ends. Transitioning occurs when someone is in the process of returning to their natural hair after permanently altering. This stage may be managed by either routinely trimming the altered ends over time or opting for a "big chop", cutting off the altered hair all at once. Because Transitioning Hair has two or more textures, each with different needs, behaviors, and responses to products and styling, it is more prone to tangling, breakage, and styling frustrations if not managed with intentional, targeted care. By recognizing "Transitioning" as its own distinct Texture State, it becomes easier to recommend appropriate products, suggest compatible styling options, and provide the emotional support many need during this unique and often sensitive phase of their hair journey. Texture State™ describes the hair's standing condition in relation to its original structure and is assessed independently of any single service. *See also: Texture Recovery™, which evaluates the hair's response to a specific service.*

### Determining Texture State

Determining Texture State is crucial because it helps eliminate assumptions and misconceptions about the hair's properties and provides a foundational reference point for discussing the hair's condition and recommended treatments and services. Here's a framework to assess whether hair is natural or altered based on its characteristics and history:

- **Explore Hair History** - Discuss with your client their past hair care routine, treatments, and chemical services (e.g., relaxers, perms, bleaching, or keratin straightening). Inquire how often and when the last time direct heat was used to straighten or stretch the hair (e.g., flat irons, curling wands, round brushing, concentrated blow-drying). And find how often and when the last time the hair was subjected to high tension, friction, or high manipulation styling (sew-in weaves, wig, extension, braid, or tight pulled-back styles). Learning this history will provide you with insight into what may be the cause of inconsistencies in texture, damage to strands, and what residual chemical treatments may still remain in the hair.

- **Thoroughly Cleanse -** To properly analyze hair's Texture State, the hair should be thoroughly cleansed from product build-up and properly conditioned so that the true condition of the hair may be visible and the true hair properties can be revealed.
- **Observation -** Examine the hair shaft, root to end, to detect any lines of demarcation that show distinct differences between the natural hair texture (normally at the new growth) and the altered hair texture (normally at the mid to ends of the hair shaft). Signs of altered texture may be observed in differences in tightness of the Texture Shape, inconsistent Texture Patterns (whether loss of pattern or a gained uniformity in pattern from a chemical curl process), or color inconsistencies. Also, look for visible damage such as frizz, breakage, or split ends that might suggest alteration. In addition, conduct a Porosity test and compare it to previous documented hair analysis to determine if a permanent change in porosity occurred. Cuticle damage often causes hair to become more porous.

**Common Assumptions & Misunderstandings**

Identifying your client's Texture State grants you the opportunity to educate your clients on the current state of their hair and how they must grow out and trim away permanently altered hair. This gives the opportunity to address a common misunderstanding that chemical processes, heat damage, and other changes can wear off hair. Another common assumption regarding the state of hair texture is that all hair that hasn't been chemically processed is in its natural state. This assumption is false: **CHEMICAL-FREE DOES NOT EQUAL NATURAL.** This is because the introduction of chemical services is not the only means of permanently altering hair. High-temperature exposure can permanently alter the natural structure of hair bonds, just as chemical processes can permanently alter hair bonds. Hair that has had its texture shape permanently altered, without chemical processing, is commonly known as **Straight Natural**.

Straight Natural refers to highly textured hair that has been permanently altered through heat exposure that surpassed the hair's heat threshold, resulting in a looser or partially relaxed texture shape. Although the texture shape changes, the hair continues to perform well across other Hair Properties, such as elasticity, porosity, strength, and other thresholds. Because the hair remains healthy, resilient, and able to thrive, this state is not classified as heat damage. Instead, Straight Natural represents a stable, altered texture state where the hair retains its overall integrity, responds predictably to care, and achieves a consistently sleek, smooth thermal press with proper servicing and care.

High-lift blonding can also permanently strip hair of its elasticity, texture, shape, and pattern, just as chemical treatments. In both scenarios, it is quite possible to permanently alter the hair without a chemical process. A third common assumption is that all hair that is not a wig, weave, or extension is natural because it grows from the scalp. This misunderstanding does not take into account the fact that hair that has grown from the scalp can be permanently altered from its natural state.

**Referencing Texture State In Consultation**

When individuals and stylists share a common understanding of Texture State, it creates a foundation for effective collaboration. One of the most important reasons to determine Texture State is to establish a clear, shared understanding of what is achievable when styling and maintaining the hair. Misunderstandings about the state of hair can lead to unmet expectations, styling challenges, and even damage. Here are ways that referencing the client's Texture State helps to provide a fundamental reference point when discussing the condition of the hair and recommending treatments and services:

- **Aligns Styling Goals with Hair's True State:** When discussing Natural Hair, you should indicate whether the client wishes to maintain the hair's original natural texture, consequently providing styling options that enhance and complement its natural texture (e.g., twist-outs, wash-and-gos, braid-outs). When working with altered hair, you should explain that altered hair may have limitations due to damage, heat, or chemical changes, necessitating styles that accommodate weakened or inconsistent textures (e.g., protective styles, heatless curls, smoothing treatments), and discuss a recommended path to restoring or trimming away the damaged hair.

- **Minimizes Styling Frustrations:** Identifying Texture State helps stylists and clients avoid missteps, ensuring that the chosen styles and home care are compatible with the hair's current state.
- **Guides Product and Tool Selection**: Different Texture States require tailored products and tools for optimal styling results. For example, Natural hair often benefits from heavier moisture-based products, while Altered Hair may require reparative treatments, smoothing serums, or heat-protectant products to support styling. Without understanding Texture State, individuals might use products or tools that don't align with their hair's needs, leading to subpar results or damage.
- **Predicts Styling Durability Expectations**: Knowing the Texture State helps set realistic timelines and expectations for how long styles will last and what maintenance they require. Styles based on the structure of natural hair (like twist-outs or wash-and-gos) tend to last longer and revert to the natural texture shape with minimal effort. Styles on Altered Hair may lack longevity or fail to revert, especially if heat or chemical damage has compromised the hair's natural elasticity.
- **Facilitates Clear Communication:** When individuals and stylists share a common understanding of Texture State, it creates a foundation for effective collaboration.
- **Builds Confidence Through Realistic Outcomes:** When clients understand their Texture State, they can confidently choose styles that highlight their hair's strengths while respecting its limitations. This prevents the emotional and physical toll of failed styling attempts or damage caused by trying to force the hair into incompatible styles.

By determining Texture State, both clients and stylists can communicate with the same understanding. This ensures that styling options and expectations are realistic, achievable, and aligned with the hair's true condition and goals. This shared understanding fosters better results, healthier hair, and greater satisfaction.

## Texture Movement™

Hair Textures are inherently dynamic. It exists in a constant state of motion as it emerges from the scalp to bend, turn, and curve to create shape and patterns. Highly textured hair, with kinks, coils, and curls, tends to have greater degrees of movement. This continuous motion is referred to as **Texture Movement**, and begins with 3 three key aspects: Angle of Emergence, Natural Fall, and Perpetual Motion.

**Angle of Emergence**: The Angle of Emergence is the general angle at which hair exits the scalp, playing a critical role in its overall texture and behavior. Straight hair

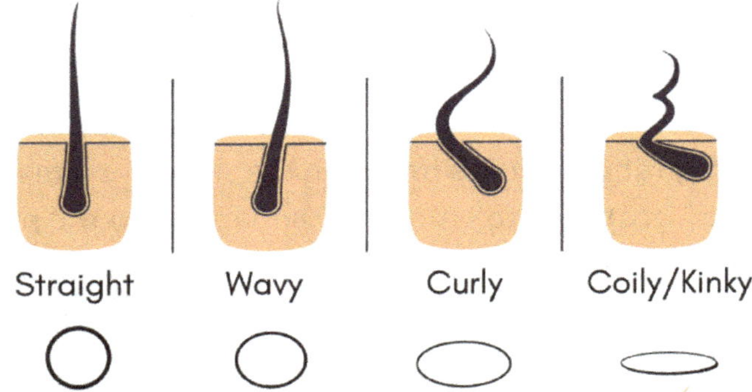


emerges at a more perpendicular angle to the scalp, contributing to its sleek, smooth appearance. In contrast, highly textured hair emerges at an angle, creating waves, curls, kinks, or coils. Angle of Emergence may also cause cowlicks, which are areas of the scalp where hair exists in opposite directions within one area, causing hair to spiral at the scalp. These varying differences influence cutting, shaping, product application, extension placement, and styling techniques, making it essential for professionals to tailor their approach based on hair growth patterns.

**Natural Fall**: Natural Fall refers to the way hair naturally positions itself in response to gravity, based on its inherent texture shape and Angle of Emergence. While straight hair tends to fall downward, maintaining a smooth and elongated form, highly textured hair exhibits multidirectional movement, growing outward, upward, downward, or diagonally. Understanding this Natural Fall is crucial in cutting, sectioning, and designing hairstyles that enhance rather than fight against the hair's intrinsic tendencies.

**Perpetual Motion**: Perpetual Motion refers to the continuous, responsive movement of hair textures as it expands, contracts, and reshapes itself in reaction to structural changes like protein loss, internal changes like vitamin deficiencies, external influences like hard water, environmental exposure like temperature fluctuations, and manipulation. Unlike straight hair, which remains relatively static in its growth direction, highly textured hair is in constant dynamic motion. More examples of hair's perpetual motion can be found in the way that highly textured hair will mat and lock if left without detangling, or how these hair textures frizz in response to humid climates. Recognizing this adaptability allows professionals to anticipate changes in hair behavior, providing informed recommendations on styling techniques, product usage, and maintenance routines that support hair health and create predictability in finished styles.

**Understanding Angle of Emergence**

The Angle of Emergence is determined by the shape of the hair follicle, which directly influences the hair's texture, movement, and overall behavior. **Round follicles** allow hair to emerge straight from the scalp with no bending or curling. This results in a lack of Texture Movement, causing the hair to fall directly downward due to gravity's pull.

**Oval follicles** produce strands that exit the scalp at a slight angle, forming waves with gentle bends. These waves tend to lie closer to the scalp and flow slightly outward and downward. As the strands grow longer, gravity may cause them to appear straighter.

**Narrow oval follicles** cause strands to emerge at an acute angle, forming curls. The flatter the follicle, the tighter the curl. These helical structures exhibit both upward and outward movement.

**Flattened oval follicles** produce strands that emerge from the scalp at an acute angle, creating kinks and coils. These tightly wound structures result in compact bends that grow upward and outward.

# Texture Movement Spectrum™

**Texture Movement Spectrum™** is the umbrella term for the full range of variable movement that hair expresses, from tightly coiled to completely straight, with every form of bend, wave, frizz, and incongruency in between. It encompasses both Texture Shape™, which describes the form and curvature of the strand, and Texture Pattern™, which describes how consistently that shape repeats along the length of the hair. Together, these two elements map not just what the hair looks like, but how it moves, responds, and behaves, providing a complete picture that curl pattern alone was never designed to deliver. The spectrum is continuous and not centered around a single texture shape, as the standard.

Describing all hair movement as a curl does a disservice to the very clarity this framework is designed to create. Curl implies a specific formation, a loop, a coil, a spiral, and by extension, it positions straight, wavy, and incongruent textures either as outliers or as absent from texture altogether. This is inaccurate. Straight hair has downward movement. Wavy hair has oscillation. Hair that is frizzy, wiry, or incongruent in its pattern has movement; it simply does not move in a way that forms a recognizable, repeating curl. The Texture Movement Spectrum corrects this by placing movement at the center of the conversation rather than curl. Every Texture Shape has a place on the spectrum, and every texture, whether consistent or incongruent, can be accurately described within it. This is not a cosmetic reframing. It is a more precise diagnostic language that serves every client, every texture, and every professional who uses it.

## Texture Shape™

**Texture Shape** refers to the form and curvature of a hair strand and where it lies within the Texture Movement Spectrum, ranging from tightly coiled to straight or frizzy. There are six Texture Shapes: kinky, coily, curly, wavy, straight, and incongruent. Each has distinct features and behavior, primarily determined by the degree of movement.

**Kinky Hair** forms tight, sharp bends and "Z" shape, often displaying a High Degree of Shrinkage that can reduce the visible length by up to 90%. However, in some cases, the zigzags may rest as a tight wave with minimal contraction, resulting in a lower degree of shrinkage, often around 50% or less.

**Coily Hair** forms tight corkscrew, helix, or "O" shaped curls. This Texture Shape has a High Degree of Shrinkage, often reducing the visible length by up to 90%. The true length of coily hair can be challenging to assess without stretching, as the hair's natural shrinkage often makes it appear significantly shorter than it actually is, even as it continues to grow.

**Curly Hair** forms spirals or loops, ranging from loose, bouncy curls to tighter ringlets, with defined "S" or "O" shapes. Curly hair often springs outward and upward, creating volume and lift. This Texture Shape has a Medium Degree of Shrinkage, up to 50% of its true length.

**Wavy Hair**, characterized by loose, flowing "S" shapes, moving in gentle undulations. Wavy hair typically lies closer to the scalp while still exhibiting visible bends. It has a Low Degree of Shrinkage (5%-30%) and can balance between oily and dry, depending on factors such as density and porosity.

**Straight Hair**, as the name suggests, lacks natural bends or curves and falls uniformly from the scalp. This texture shape moves freely and fluidly, often appearing sleek and shiny due to its ability to reflect light. Straight hair typically experiences no shrinkage.

**Incongruent Texture Shape** refers to hair that bends and curves in primarily frizzy or wiry movement without a distinct curl or wave formation, and often appears unruly. Wiry hair is normally a result of natural greying, medication, thermal styling, and excessive manipulation. Depleted or distressed hair may also have an Incongruent

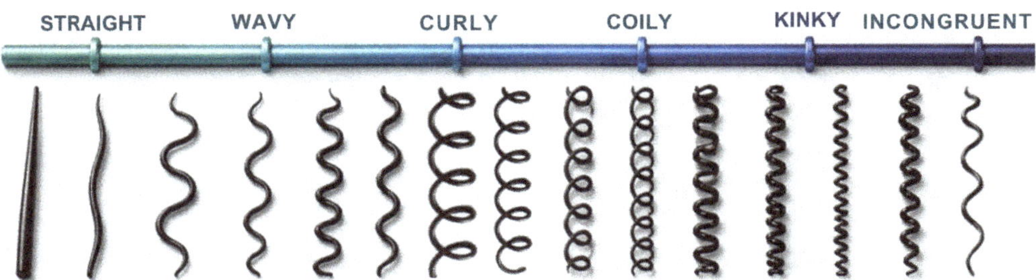

Texture Shape as a result of wearing wigs, braids, weaves, aggressive stretching, and Banding.

Each texture shape plays a significant role in determining hair care needs, product application, and styling techniques. Understanding these textures is crucial for developing effective hair care routines and managing hair's unique characteristics.

## Texture Pattern™

It is a common misconception that all hair that experiences shrinkage automatically has a curl pattern. While many individuals with highly textured hair do have clearly identifiable curls or waves, others present different forms of texture, such as frizzy, wiry, or incongruent patterns that do not conform to a uniform curl shape up and down the hair strand.

**Texture Patterns** represent how the Texture Shape repeats along the length of the hair strand. Although the terms hair texture and curl pattern are closely related concepts, they are distinct and should not be used interchangeably. Texture Patterns can be classified into two main categories:

- **Curl Patterns**: When the Texture Shape remains consistent along the length of the strand, forming a repeating, recognizable pattern of curls, waves, or coils.
- **Incongruent Textures™**: When the Texture Shape lacks consistency or repetition along the strand, displaying no discernible pattern at all.

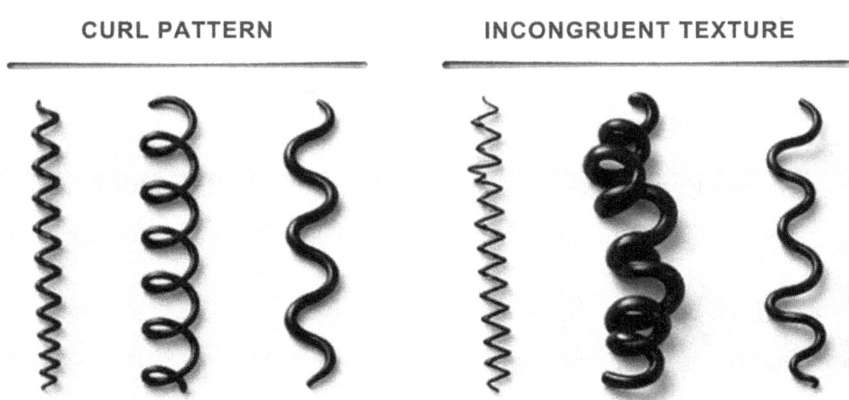

Recognizing these differences is essential for selecting appropriate hair care products, style potential, styling techniques, and maintenance strategies.

**Curly Hair** forms spirals or loops, ranging from loose, bouncy curls to tighter ringlets, with defined "S" or "O" shapes. Curly hair often springs outward and upward, creating volume and lift. This Texture Shape has a Medium Degree of Shrinkage, up to 50% of its true length.

**Wavy Hair**, characterized by loose, flowing "S" shapes, moving in gentle undulations. Wavy hair typically lies closer to the scalp while still exhibiting visible bends. It has a Low Degree of Shrinkage (5%-30%) and can balance between oily and dry, depending on factors such as density and porosity.

**Straight Hair**, as the name suggests, lacks natural bends or curves and falls uniformly from the scalp. This texture shape moves freely and fluidly, often appearing sleek and shiny due to its ability to reflect light. Straight hair typically experiences no shrinkage.

**Incongruent Texture Shape™** refers to hair that bends and curves with no distinct pattern throughout the hair strand, primarily frizzy or wiry movement without a distinct curl or wave formation and often appears unruly. Wiry hair is normally a result of natural greying, medication, thermal styling, and excessive manipulation. Depleted or distressed hair may also have an Incongruent Texture Shape as a result of wearing wigs, braids, weaves, aggressive stretching, and Banding.

Each texture shape plays a significant role in determining hair care needs, product application, and styling techniques. Understanding these textures is crucial for developing effective hair care routines and managing hair's unique characteristics.

## Texture Feel™ - The Fabric of Hair

**Texture Feel** refers to the tactile feel and appearance of hair. The Texture Feel of hair is shaped by a mix of genetic factors, tactile qualities, and structural composition, such as porosity, elasticity, and curl shape. Some common descriptions of the Feel of Texture Feel are:

- **Smooth:** This Texture Feel has a tightly aligned cuticle layer, resulting in a sleek, even surface with minimal friction. This type of hair often reflects light well, giving it a shiny appearance. Common structural characteristics include Low Porosity, Medium to High Elasticity, and it is often associated with straight, wavy or loosely curly hair.
- **Soft:** This Texture Feel has a fine, delicate, lightweight quality, a chiffon or velvety feel, and a matte appearance. It commonly has structural characteristics of Medium to High Porosity and medium to Low Elasticity, and is often found in curly and coily texture shapes. This Texture is normally easy to manipulate and requires frequent reshaping of set styles.
- **Silky**: It combines smoothness and softness to create a satiny feel with minimal frizz. Common structural characteristics include low porosity and medium to high elasticity, and it is often associated with straight, wavy, or loose curls.
- **Cottony:** This Texture Feel has a fine, delicate, lightweight quality with a cottony feel. Hair is fluffy and voluminous, with a soft yet slightly dry feel, with a matte appearance. Common structural characteristics include Medium to High Porosity, Medium to Low Elasticity, and is frequently found in coily or kinky hair, where compact texture shapes create a light, airy feel.
- **Wiry**: This Texture Feel has a coarse, firm, and slightly rigid feel. It often has a rough surface due to its thicker diameter and raised cuticle layers. This texture feel covers a wide range of structural characteristics, including Low to High Porosity, Low to Medium Elasticity, and is associated with straight, wavy, or loose curls. This hair is often very resistant and is less pliable.
- **Woolly**: This Texture Feel has dense, tightly entwined hair, resembling natural wool. It is often coarse and dry, with a unique thickness. Common structural characteristics include High Porosity, Mid to Low Elasticity, and are predominantly found amongst kinky or highly coily textures.

Genetic factors, environmental conditions, hair care practices, and hormonal changes can strongly influence the Texture Feel. Understanding these underlying causes allows professionals to recommend personalized care and styling solutions that complement the natural texture of the hair.

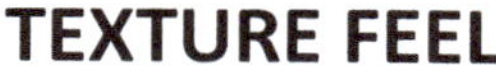


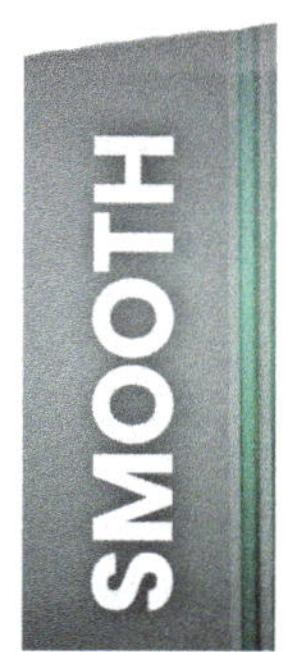


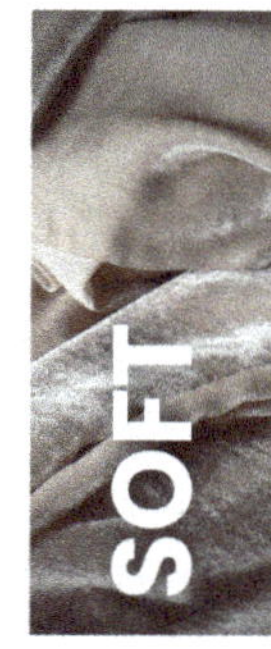


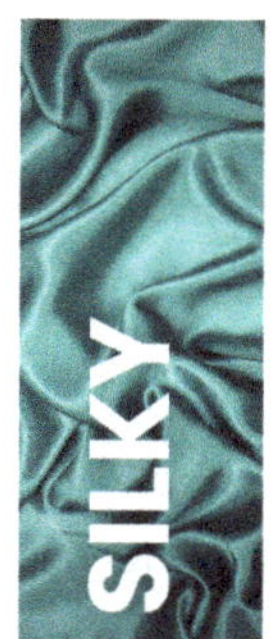


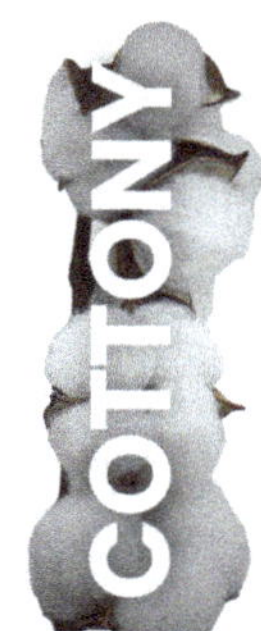


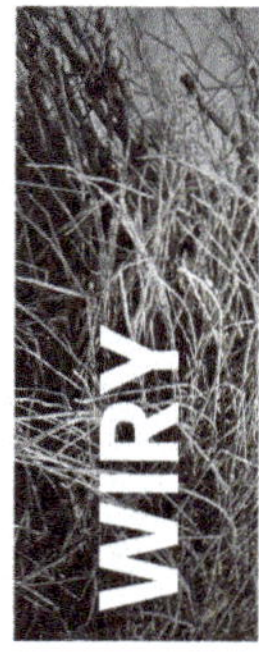


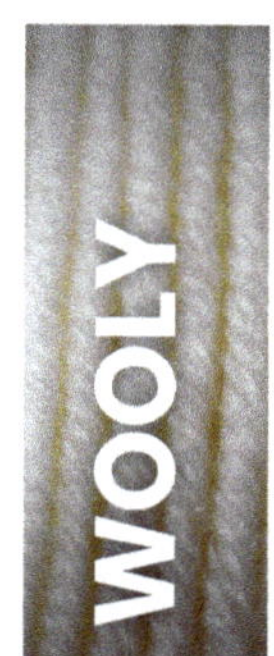


These factors include:

1. **Cuticle Structure and Alignment**:
   Hair that feels smooth, soft, or silky often has a tightly aligned cuticle layer. This allows light to reflect evenly and creates a luster and shine. Conversely, hair with raised or uneven cuticle layers may feel rough, wiry, or woolly due to its higher friction and reduced light reflection.

2. **Hair Strand Diameter**:
   The Strand Diameter plays a significant role in how hair feels. Fine hair tends to feel softer due to its smaller diameter and more pliable structure. Coarse hair, with its larger diameter, is often perceived as wiry or woolly because it is less flexible and has a more robust texture.

3. **Cortex Composition**:
   The cortex is composed of keratin proteins and moisture-binding lipids. A higher lipid-to-protein ratio contributes to softer, silkier hair, while a lower ratio or high protein content can create a more rigid, wiry texture. The specific keratin structure and distribution of sulfur bonds in the cortex also influence flexibility and softness.

4. **Sebum Production**:
   Genetics determines the amount and consistency of sebum, the natural oil produced by the scalp. Adequate sebum evenly coats the hair, making it feel soft, smooth, and silky. In contrast, hair that lacks sufficient sebum may feel dry, rough, or cottony.

5. **Texture Movement Spectrum**:
   Straighter hair tends to feel smoother and silkier due to its uniform surface. Tightly coiled or zigzag-shaped hair can feel woolly or cottony as the bends and twists disrupt the alignment of the cuticle scales.
6. **Genetic Ethnic Variations**:
   Genetic heritage influences the natural balance of hair's structural proteins and lipids, contributing to variations in texture. For example, individuals with African ancestry often have hair that feels cottony or woolly due to tightly coiled curls and less sebum distribution along the hair shaft. In contrast, hair from Asian ancestry often feels silky and smooth due to a round follicle shape and tightly compacted cuticle layers.

Each of these characteristics is shaped by the integration of genetic factors, tactile qualities, and structural composition, creating a unique fingerprint for every individual's hair.

## Key Terms

**Texture Indicators™**: The various hair characteristics that interact and work together to influence the Hair Texture.

**Texture State™**: The classification of hair's current condition in relation to its original structure

**Natural Hair™**: Hair that retains its original structure and characteristics.

**Altered Hair™**: Hair that has undergone a permanent change to its natural structure.

**Transitioning Hair™**: Hair in a mixed state, where natural texture is growing at the roots, but altered hair remains on the ends.

**Straight Natural™**: Hair that has had its texture shape permanently altered without exposure to chemicals, normally through thermal straightening.

**Texture Movement™**: Hair's constant state of motion as it emerges from the scalp to bend, turn, and curve to create shape and patterns.

**Angle of Emergence™**: The general angle at which hair exits the scalp.

**Natural Fall™**: The way hair naturally positions itself in response to gravity based on its inherent Texture Shape and Angle of Emergence.

**Perpetual Motion™**: The continuous, responsive movement of hair as it expands, contracts, and reshapes itself.

**Texture Movement Spectrum™**: The full range of variable movement that hair expresses, from tightly coiled to completely straight and incongruent, encompassing Texture Shape™ and Texture Pattern™, with no single texture as the default.

**Texture Shape™**: The form and curvature of a hair strand and where it lies within the Texture Movement Spectrum™, ranging from tightly coiled to straight or frizzy.

**Kinky Hair™**: Hair with tight, sharp bends and zigzag forms.

**Coily Hair**: Hair with tight corkscrew, helix, or "O" shaped curls.

**Curly Hair**: Hair with spirals or loops, ranging from loose, bouncy curls to tighter ringlets, with defined "S" or "O" shapes

**Wavy Hair**: Hair that is characterized by loose, flowing "S" shapes, moving in gentle undulations.

**Straight Hair**: Hair that lacks natural bends or curves and falls uniformly from the scalp.

**Incongruent Texture Shape™**: Hair that bends and curves in primarily frizzy or wiry movement without a distinct curl or wave formation, and often appears unruly.

**Texture Pattern™**: Represents how the Texture Shape repeats along the length of the hair strand.

**Curl Pattern™**: When the Texture Shape is consistent and uniform along the length of the hair.

**Incongruent Texture Pattern™**: When the Texture Shape lacks consistency or repetition along the strand, displaying no discernible pattern at all

**Texture Feel™**: The tactile feel and appearance of hair

# Texture Dynamics - Pillar 3
# HAIR TRESHOLDS™
## HAIR LIMITS & SENSITIVITIES

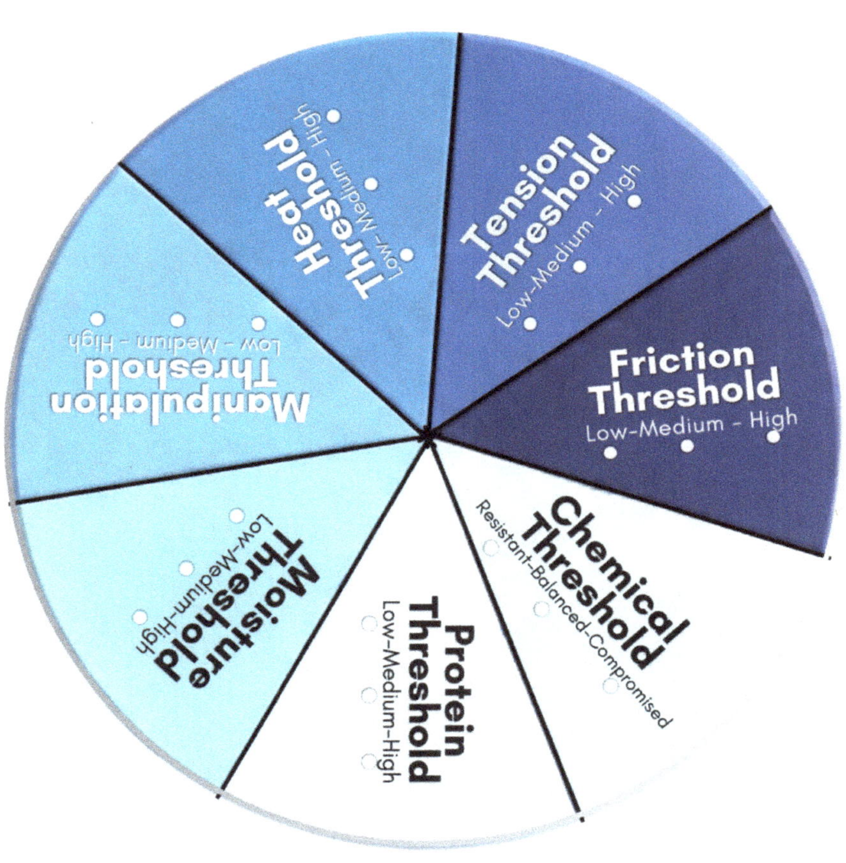

# 5.
# Pillar 3 - Hair Thresholds™

*The limits of tolerance that hair has.*

**Hair Thresholds**™ represent the limits of tolerance that hair has for various external stressors and internal variances encountered during styling, hair care, and treatment practices. Multiple thresholds must be considered as they significantly affect hair's overall health and resilience. There are six main Hair Thresholds, including:

- Protein Threshold™
- Moisture Threshold™
- Heat Threshold™
- Chemical Threshold™
- Manipulation Threshold™
- Tension Threshold™
- Friction Threshold™

Each threshold differs from person to person and is influenced by factors such as hair's natural structure, hair history, and environmental exposure.
*View Threshold Diagnostic Tables - See Appendix.*

Unlike Pillars 1 and 2, which can be assessed in a single session, Pillar 3 is built through ongoing tracking of the hair's behavior. To accurately assess these thresholds, cosmetologists should observe and document the hair's response to these various stressors. This assessment provides a comprehensive profile that reflects the hair's unique needs and capabilities. Equipped with this information, professionals can make targeted, customized recommendations, so specific reparative treatments, protective styles, or styling techniques, and home care can be recommended.

This detailed, personalized approach ensures that each client's hair is not only understood but also nurtured in a way that supports its natural texture, strengths, weaknesses, and long-term health. Over time, this leads to improved hair resilience, better style retention, and increased confidence for the client.

# Protein Thresholds™

**Protein Threshold** refers to the maximum amount of protein your hair can absorb before it starts to experience adverse effects. Hair exhibits varying levels of tolerance to protein, determining how much protein reinforcement the hair can accept before its integrity is compromised, and it is closely influenced by factors such as low porosity, strand diameter, and overall fiber condition. *View Threshold Diagnostic Tables - See Appendix.*

Hair with a **Low Protein Threshold** often tends to have lower porosity. It already has a natural strength to it and doesn't need a lot of extra protein reinforcement. If you add too much, it can begin feeling stiff and brittle. The cuticle structure is compact, limiting protein absorption and minimizing structural weaknesses, which means protein treatments should be used sparingly and with caution.

**Medium Protein Threshold** hair falls within a moderate range of porosity and elasticity. This hair type can comfortably tolerate a balanced regimen of protein and moisture, making it relatively resilient under routine care. It does not exhibit an extreme response to the addition or lack of routine protein treatments.

**High Protein Threshold** is often associated with high porosity hair, maybe coarser or more porous hair, or hair that has experienced structural wear from environmental, chemical, or mechanical stress. These strands tend to benefit greatly from routine protein treatments, as the raised or damaged cuticle allows for increased protein penetration. Ongoing reinforcement helps maintain structural integrity and elasticity, reducing the risk of breakage.

In general, the lower the porosity, the lower the hair's protein threshold; the higher the porosity, the greater the need for regular protein support. Medium-porosity hair falls between these two ends of the spectrum and requires a more flexible, balanced approach to protein application.

Understanding hair porosity and its relationship with protein tolerance is key to proper hair care. High-porosity hair generally benefits from protein due to its structural weaknesses, while low-porosity hair requires protein more sparingly. Additionally, different types of proteins affect the hair differently; larger proteins like keratin and collagen form a film on the hair, while smaller hydrolyzed proteins penetrate the shaft, making it crucial to choose products based on hair needs.

## Moisture Thresholds™

**Moisture Threshold** refers to the maximum level of hydration or moisture loss that hair can withstand without compromising its structural integrity. It's not just how much moisture hair can "take in", it's also how much fluctuation of intake and loss it can handle before weakening, swelling, or breaking. Every individual has a unique Moisture Threshold, which is influenced by hair porosity, hair care routine, lifestyle, physical health, and environmental exposure. When hair remains within this threshold, it is flexible, pliable, and resilient. However, exceeding or falling below this threshold leads to a range of moisture-related hair issues.

Moisture Threshold can be categorized into three levels: high, medium, and low, based on how it responds to moisture fluctuations and how well it maintains structural integrity when exposed to hydration or moisture loss. Understanding these thresholds allows stylists and clients to make informed decisions about product selection, layering, and regimen design. *View Threshold Diagnostic Tables - See Appendix.*

**High Moisture Threshold hair** often includes low-porosity strands with tightly layered cuticles and strong elasticity. This hair type is slow to absorb moisture and equally slow to lose it. It can tolerate wide swings in moisture exposure (from dryness to deep hydration) without breaking down easily. However, it typically requires extended hydration time or the use of mild heat to allow moisture to penetrate the strand. It's also vulnerable to product buildup, especially when heavy, occlusive products are layered unnecessarily. The best product strategy is to use lightweight hydrators, mild humectants, and gentle heat to support absorption, while avoiding heavy layers that won't absorb well.

**Medium Moisture Threshold hair** typically exhibits moderate porosity and elasticity. This hair type absorbs and retains moisture relatively easily, without the need for intensive effort. It maintains hydration for several days and responds well to standard moisturizing routines. A balanced regimen that combines hydrating products with a light-to-moderate sealing product is typically effective. This group benefits from regular moisture maintenance without extremes in either direction.

**Low Moisture Threshold hair** is commonly associated with high-porosity strands, in which the cuticle layer is raised or damaged, and elasticity is reduced. This hair absorbs moisture very quickly but also loses it just as fast, which makes it highly vulnerable to overhydration and hygral fatigue. While it often seems like this hair needs lots of moisture, too much rewetting or heavy hydrating products can actually weaken it. The best approach is to use rich, occlusive products that seal in moisture effectively and minimize unnecessary saturation between wash days.

## Tailored Strategies for Each Threshold Level

Hair with **High Moisture Threshold** benefits most from mild heat or steam during hydration to gently lift the cuticle and allow moisture to penetrate. Hydration should be applied in layers, with a focus on lightweight products to avoid buildup. Heavy creams, butters, and oils should be used sparingly and only when the hair is exceptionally dry.

For hair with **Medium Moisture Threshold,** the ideal regimen is a balanced and uncomplicated routine. Alternate between moisturizing and strengthening treatments to keep the hair healthy and resilient. Light-to-moderate sealing oils are usually sufficient to lock in moisture without overwhelming the strand.

Hair with **Low Moisture Threshold** should be treated with rich, occlusive products immediately after hydration to prevent rapid moisture loss. Frequent saturation and over-moisturizing should be avoided, as this can weaken the hair fiber. Prioritize bond-repair and cuticle-reinforcing treatments to support the hair's structure and reduce porosity-related vulnerabilities.

## Moisture Management

Although often used interchangeably, hydration, moisturization, and sealants serve different but complementary roles in maintaining healthy hair. **Hydration** is the process of increasing the water content of the hair using water or water-based products, such as conditioners, leave-ins, and mists. These agents penetrate the hair shaft, soften the hair, and temporarily swell the cuticle, thereby increasing elasticity. Ingredients known as humectants, including glycerin, aloe vera, and honey, play a crucial role in this process by attracting and binding water to the hair, ensuring deeper hydration.

While hydration involves increasing the hair's water content, **Moisturization** is the process of maintaining that hydration by using emollients and conditioners that contain both water and oil. This step acts as a binder, helping slow hydration loss. The water component reconnects with the hydration already present in the hair, while the oils in the moisturizer connect to added oil that may be added to help form a sealant. Think of moisturization as the "middle layer" that stabilizes and extends the life of hydration, sealing it in.

This keeps hair soft, pliable, and smooth. Moisturization typically comes from creams, milks, or leave-ins that are water-based but enhanced with light oils, humectants, and film-formers. Additionally, deep conditioning treatments are effective in restoring internal moisture levels, helping to replenish and maintain moisture over time. Without proper moisturization, hydration is temporary, and the hair can quickly dry out.

**Sealants** are hydrophobic (water-repelling) substances applied to the outer surface of the hair to create a protective barrier over the hair shaft, preventing moisture loss caused by evaporation and environmental factors. This ensures the hair remains nourished and hydrated for longer periods. Common occlusives include oils and butters, such as shea butter, coconut oil, and grapeseed oil. Sealants don't moisturize the hair; they preserve the moisture that's already there.

Hydration quenches the hair's thirst by replenishing its internal water content, while moisturization supports that hydration by helping the hair retain moisture for extended periods, creating a balanced and flexible structure. Sealants complete the moisture cycle by forming a protective barrier around the hair shaft, locking in hydration and shielding the cuticle from environmental stress and moisture loss. Together, these three steps ensure the hair remains supple, resilient, and consistently nourished..

**How to Determine Current Moisture Levels™**

**Moisture Levels™** in hair refer to the amount of water content that the hair strands hold. Three key moisture levels to look out for include,

**Moisture Levels™**

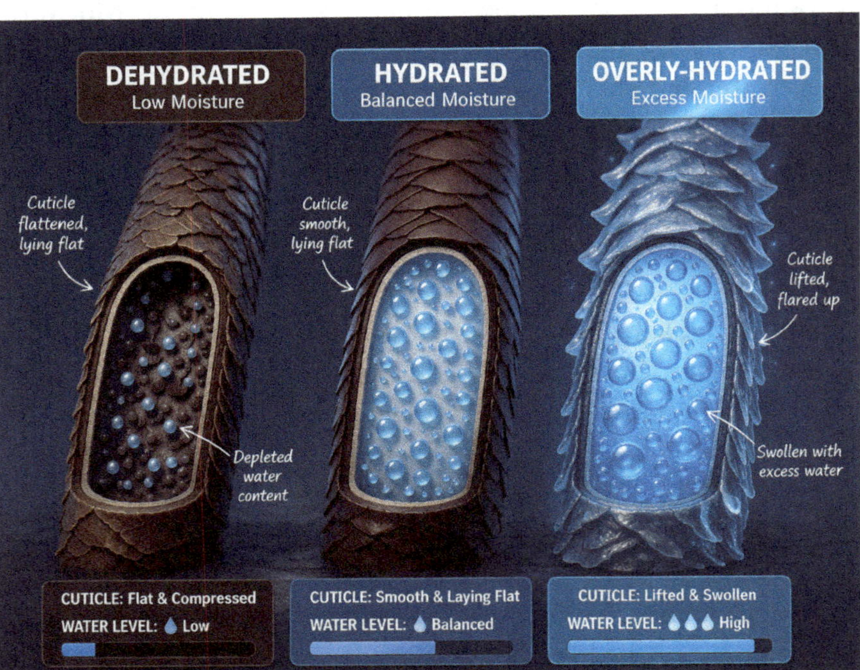


- **Hydrated (Optimal Moisture Level)**
  Hair is fully hydrated and moisturized and contains an optimal amount of water. At this level, the hair retains elasticity, pliability, and suppleness.
- **Dehydrated (Low Moisture Level)**
  Dehydrated hair is extremely dry and lacks both moisture and essential oils. It may feel lifeless, brittle, and straw-like, and curls may lose their definition

completely. Dehydration can occur from overuse of heat styling tools, environmental stress, harsh chemical treatments, or not replenishing moisture regularly. This is the most severe level of moisture loss and can result in significant hair damage if not addressed.

- **Overly Hydrated (Excessive Moisture Level)**
  When hair has experienced excessive hydration, it may develop hygral fatigue, resulting in swelling and lifting of the cuticles. This is experienced as a mushy or gummy feel, excessive elasticity, or loss of resilience.

To accurately assess a client's moisture level, begin with a porosity and behavior test. Mist a clean, dry section of the hair and observe the water's reaction. If the water beads up and sits on top of the hair, this suggests a **high moisture threshold**, commonly associated with **low porosity**, where the tightly packed cuticles resist absorption. On the other hand, if the water soaks in immediately and the hair dries quickly, the strand likely has a **low moisture threshold**, often associated with **high porosity**, in which moisture enters and escapes the hair fiber rapidly.

Next, perform an elasticity check by gently stretching a wet strand. If the strand snaps quickly without stretching, the hair may be at a low moisture level. If it stretches significantly before breaking, but does not return to its original curl shape, it may be over-hydrated, indicating that the hair is retaining too much moisture and may be vulnerable to hygral fatigue.

Lastly, monitor how long the hair stays hydrated between wash days. Hair with a **high moisture threshold** typically maintains its hydration longer, though it may take more time or effort to achieve full hydration. This behavior over time helps confirm the strand's capacity for moisture retention and tolerance.

## Hygral Fatigue

**Hygral Fatigue** is commonly recognized in the "natural hair" community as a phenomenon where hair weakens due to repeated swelling and contraction from excessive hydration. While this concept has not been extensively backed by scientific research, the absence of formal studies does not invalidate the real-world experiences of individuals who notice changes in their hair following excessive hydration and moisture treatments. Common signs of Hygral Fatigue include hair that is overly soft and limp, increased frizz, extreme weakness when wet, excessive tangling, breakage, lack of longevity in styles, and difficulty maintaining styles.

On the other hand, when hair lacks sufficient moisture, it becomes brittle, loses elasticity, and is more susceptible to breakage. Signs of insufficient moisture include a rough, coarse, or stiff texture, increased tangling due to a lack of slip, a higher tendency for breakage and split ends, undefined and frizzy curls, and a dull, lackluster appearance.

Moisture balance in hair is influenced by several factors, including external conditions, hair care regimen, and hair structure. External factors such as hard water, weather, sun exposure, and humidity levels play a significant role. High humidity can cause hair to absorb excessive moisture, leading to limpness and frizz, while low humidity can strip hair of moisture, resulting in dry, brittle hair. Water quality affects moisture retention, as hard water deposits minerals on the hair, making it more difficult for moisture to penetrate. Additionally, humectants like glycerin can either help retain moisture in humid conditions or pull moisture from the hair in dry climates, exacerbating dryness.
Regarding product usage and hair care routines, overusing moisturizing products such as leave-ins, deep conditioners, or co-washing treatments can lead to excessive hydration, which can weaken the hair over time. Another key factor is a lack of protein balance, as hair requires both moisture and protein. Too much moisture without adequate protein can leave hair weak and fragile. Additionally, improper product layering, such as applying heavy sealants before hydrating products, can prevent moisture from being properly absorbed.

Hair structure itself determines how moisture is retained. High-porosity hair absorbs and loses moisture quickly, making it prone to dehydration if not properly sealed, while low-porosity hair has difficulty absorbing moisture in the first place. Texture and density also play a role, as finer strands reach their moisture threshold more quickly than coarser hair, requiring careful product selection to avoid overloading or drying out the hair. Understanding these factors can help maintain optimal moisture balance, keeping hair healthy and resilient.

Maintaining the right moisture balance in hair requires regular assessment and adjustments based on its condition and environment. Pay close attention to how your hair feels. If it becomes too soft and weak, incorporating protein treatments can help strengthen it, while stiffness and dryness indicate a need for increased hydration. Using protein-moisture balancing products is essential for maintaining structural integrity while keeping hair properly hydrated. Additionally, adjusting your routine based on environmental conditions can prevent moisture-related issues; for example, reducing humectant use in dry climates and relying more on sealants can help prevent excessive moisture loss, while increasing humectants in humid conditions can enhance hydration.

## Moisture Cycle™

The **Moisture Cycle** for hair is the natural process by which hair absorbs, retains, and loses moisture over time. Highly textured hair tends to be naturally dry because its bent, curved, or coiled structure makes it harder for the scalp's natural oils to travel down the strands. This is why they require moisture, but also why it loses it faster than straight hair. Here's what happens in the moisture cycle: On wash day, your curls are at their most hydrated after cleansing and conditioning, setting the foundation for your moisture level. During standard days two and three, the moisture begins to evaporate, and curls may feel drier and lose definition. By mid-week, frizz and tangling may increase, and the hair might look dull or lifeless without replenishment. By day seven and beyond, the hair will feel drier, less defined, and more prone to breakage.

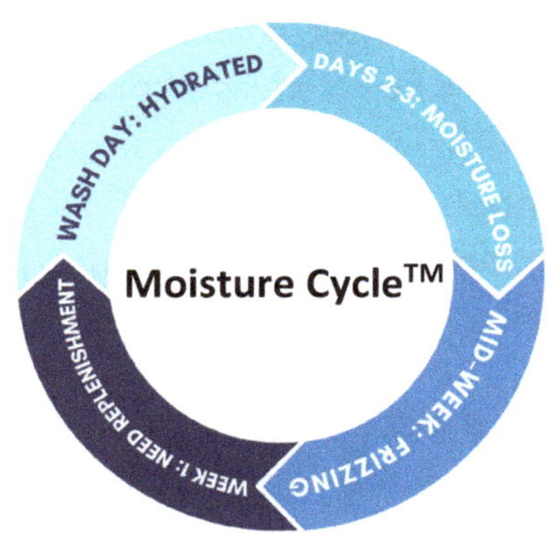


## Moisture Retention Regimen™

A **Moisture Retention Regimen** involves a routine of layering hydrators and moisturizers to maintain a healthy moisture level throughout the Moisture Cycle. The three types of hydrations include: hydrators, sealants, and refreshers that work together to keep curls moisturized and resistant to dryness and breakage, ensuring hydration is sustained between wash days. The first layer of hydrators infuses the hair with water-based hydration to replenish the internal hydration level. This can be achieved using leave-in conditioners, moisturizing hair mists, and hydrating sprays that contain humectants like glycerin, aloe vera, honey, sodium PCA, and propanediol. These ingredients attract and bind water to the hair, helping it retain moisture. Additionally, hydrolyzed proteins such as silk protein, wheat protein, keratin, and collagen reinforce the hair's structure, improving its ability to hold water. Panthenol (Pro-Vitamin B5) also plays a dual role, acting as both a humectant and emollient to smooth and strengthen the hair cuticle.

Once hydration is introduced, the second layer provides moisturization, which involves sealing in the hydration to prevent rapid evaporation with products that have a water and oil emulsion. This layer consists of a water-based emulsion with emollients like shea butter, cocoa butter, coconut oil, avocado oil, and jojoba oil. At times, a single oil may be used as a one-step sealant. These ingredients seal in moisture while smoothing the cuticle, making hair feel soft and reducing friction and breakage. Fatty alcohols such as cetearyl, stearyl, and behenyl alcohol are often added to provide. Additionally, ceramides and phospholipids help reinforce the hair's natural lipid barrier, further preventing moisture loss and supporting elasticity.

As the moisture cycle continues, leading to the next wash day, hair gradually loses moisture due to environmental exposure, manipulation, and natural evaporation. To maintain hydration, a refresher should be used to reactivate moisture without causing buildup. This layer includes moisture-refreshing sprays, scalp and hair conditioning mists, and lightweight hydrating serums. Ingredients such as aloe vera and rose water provide lightweight hydration, while hydrolyzed silk or rice protein helps reinforce the hair cuticle to maintain hydration balance.

These three layers work together to ensure long-lasting moisture retention. The hydration layer introduces water-based moisture, the moisturization layer locks it in to prevent excessive loss, and the refreshing layer helps maintain moisture levels throughout the week. By following this Moisture Retention Regimen, curls remain nourished, resilient, and well-moisturized, effectively supporting the hair's natural moisture cycle and reducing the need for frequent rehydration.

The benefits of maintaining the moisture level through the moisture cycle include

- **Length Retention**: Proper moisture prevents dryness and breakage by keeping hair pliable.
- **Manageability**: Well-moisturized hair resists tangling and frizz, making it easier to detangle and style.
- **Expanded Styling Options**: Hydrated hair holds styles better, whether it's smooth, straight looks, or defined curls.

## Heat Threshold™

The **Heat Threshold** refers to the point at which hair can no longer endure thermal exposure without experiencing structural changes and possibly compromising its overall health. Heat Threshold Levels represent a scale of how much thermal exposure hair can withstand, ranging from low to high. Factors like porosity, strand diameter, moisture balance, hair history, and overall health influence these levels. Unfortunately, Heat Threshold Levels can often only be determined after the hair has experienced irreversible change and then noted for future thermal exposure. *View Threshold Diagnostic Tables - See Appendix.*

**Low Heat Threshold hair** typically includes fine strands, high-porosity fibers, dehydrated hair, and hair that has been chemically treated or color-processed. This type of hair is easily compromised by heat, often losing its texture shape and elasticity, and feeling dry, brittle, or fragile after exposure. **Medium Heat Threshold hair** generally includes Medium Diameter Strands, moderate Porosity, and often untreated natural texture. It can tolerate occasional heat styling when proper precautions are taken, such as using a heat protectant and moderate temperatures. **High Heat Threshold hair** often includes Thick Diameter Strands with Low Porosity and strong Elasticity. While this type of hair is more resilient and can handle higher levels of heat, it still requires thoughtful care to avoid cumulative damage over time. Medium to High Threshold hair is often capable of being heat trained without experiencing damage to the integrity of the hair.

To build a heat-conscious regimen, strategies should align with the hair's threshold level. For **Low Heat Threshold hair**, direct heat should be avoided or limited to one or two times per year with a great deal of heat protection and pre-treatment with steam conditioning to build the strand interior. When heat is used, temperatures should not exceed 300°F, and exposure should be brief, with no more than 1 pass of the thermal styling tool. This hair responds best to protein-rich treatments, leave-ins with thermal protection, and bonding agents that reinforce internal structure. For **Medium Heat Threshold hair**, occasional heat use is typically safe. Temperatures between 300°F and 350°F are appropriate, as long as pass-throughs are even and controlled. This hair benefits from thermal protectants and restorative deep conditioners after heat styling. For **High Heat Threshold hair**, more frequent heat use may be tolerated, with temperatures ranging from 350°F to 400°F. However, excessive passes should still be avoided. Optimal products for this group include strengthening masks and oils with high smoke points, such as grapeseed or argan oil.

It's important to remember that heat thresholds can vary across different areas of the scalp. What the crown can tolerate may differ from the crown area. And just because hair appears to "handle" heat well doesn't mean frequent use is harmless. The ultimate goal is to work *with* your hair's threshold, not against it, by using heat intentionally and protectively to preserve long-term health and texture integrity.

## Levels of Heat Response™

**Heat Response™** is the spectrum of thermal behaviors hair may experience in response to heat exposure. Hair responds to:

- How the heat is delivered
- How concentrated it is
- Whether moisture is present or removed

Low to moderate heat temporarily softens hair bonds, allowing hair to be reshaped, but excessive heat can denature keratin proteins, permanently weakening the hair and altering its natural texture shape. High heat can also destroy disulfide bonds, which are responsible for the hair's natural texture shape, resulting in limp or uneven curls. Additionally, heat exposure can

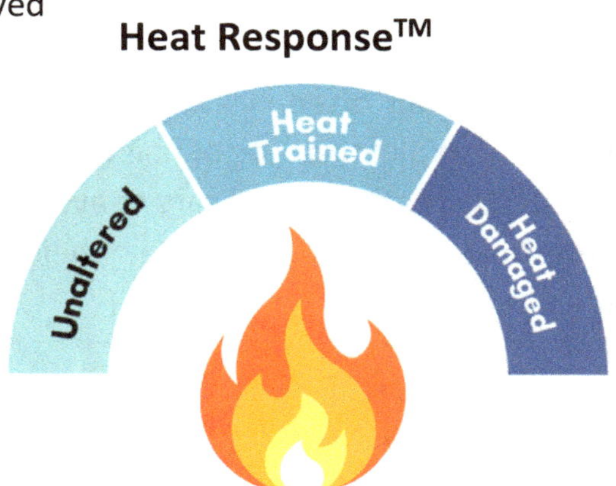

of hair textures, one must begin to see heat not as a singular force, but as a spectrum of thermal behaviors. There are 5 ways that heat is administered to hair:

- Atmospheric Heat
- Direct Heat
- Steam Heat
- Radiant Heat
- Ionic Influenced Heat

**Atmospheric Heat™** is the distribution of heat into the atmosphere surrounding the hair, i.e., Hooded and Bonnet Dryers. By administering heat in a way that envelops the hair rather than directly targeting sections at a time, the intensity of heat exposure lessens, water gradually evaporates, and heat wraps around the hair more evenly and with greater control. As a result, the texture shape is allowed to remain largely undisturbed. The hair dries within its set formation, making this type of heat particularly suitable for wet sets, molding, and styles that rely on shape preservation. Hair with a Low Heat Threshold best thrives with Atmospheric Heat.

**Direct Heat™** is the immediate transfer of heat from the heat source to the hair's surface. Here, heat is transferred through direct contact between a blow-dryer nozzle and the hair, or between flat irons, curling irons, and hot combs and the hair. Because of this, conductive heat holds the greatest potential for both refinement and risk and should be reserved for healthy hair with Medium to High Heat Thresholds. Direct heat does not inherently damage the hair, but it does initiate change. In controlled conditions, it can create smoothness, uniformity, and precision. But when misaligned with the hair's thresholds, it can compromise structural integrity, leading to permanent disruption of the pattern. This is where the line between heat training and heat damage becomes most visible.

**Steam Heat™**

Unlike other forms of heat that seek to remove moisture, steam heat operates in the opposite direction. **Steam Heat** introduces warmth alongside water vapor, allowing the hair to expand rather than contract. The cuticle gently lifts, not under stress, but through hydration. Steam does not impose structure; it makes the hair more receptive and increases elasticity. This form of heat is particularly beneficial in conditioning processes, where the goal is not to alter the texture shape but to restore flexibility, softness, and internal balance. Steam Heat benefits all Heat Thresholds. However, it is important to consider that over-steaming or using steam on already over-moisturized hair can cause hygral fatigue.

**Radiant Heat™**, or infrared heat, moves beyond the surface of the hair for increased penetration by warming the hair from within. Thermal tools like infrared flat irons and tools with infrared technology use internal heating to create a more even heat distribution, potentially reducing surface-level stress when properly controlled. However, the depth of penetration also requires a greater level of awareness. Radiant heat represents a more advanced interaction, penetrating the cortex rather than sitting on the surface. This allows more resistant hair, hair with a higher strand diameter, and hair with a fragile cuticle layer to experience gradual, controlled heat with fewer passes. Controlled Radiant Heat benefits all Heat Thresholds at moderate heat levels.

Ionic technology is often misunderstood as a form of heat, but in truth, it modifies how heat behaves. **Ionic Influenced Heat™** involves applying heat while releasing negative ions to break water molecules into smaller particles. Ionic blow-dryers, brushes, and other thermal styling tools help water evaporate more efficiently, allow the cuticle to lie flatter, and make hair appear smoother with less frizz. Ionic influence does not alter the heat's temperature; it enhances how it interacts and is most beneficial for low-porosity, dense, resistant, and frizzy hair. Controlled Ionic Influenced Heat best benefits Medium to High Heat Thresholds at moderate heat levels.

When the distinction between these heat distributions is understood, the conversation about heat begins to shift. The question is no longer whether heat is good or bad because the same heat that preserves one head of hair may compromise another. The question becomes, "What type of heat is being applied, and how does it align with the hair's thresholds?" Because hair does not respond universally. Hair responds in ways that reflect its characteristics, such as elasticity, porosity, moisture balance, and structural resilience.

When the method of heat application does not correspond with the needs and limits of the hair, the result is often unintended alteration. But when heat is chosen with the intention to align with the hair's natural behavior, it becomes a tool of refinement rather than disruption. Understanding this means heat is no longer something to fear. It becomes something to master.

- Allow the hair to cool completely before touching or manipulating it to help set the style and minimize frizz.
- Limit thermal styling to no more than once a week to prevent cumulative structural damage.
- Schedule regular trims to remove split ends and support healthy hair growth and appearance.

- **Long-Term Hair Health Maintenance:**
  - Alternate between thermal styles and heat-free options, such as braid-outs, twist-outs, or roller sets, to minimize repeated heat exposure.
  - Protect the hair overnight by using silk or satin pillowcases or bonnets to reduce friction and moisture loss.
  - Consistently monitor the hair's behavior, noting any signs of reduced elasticity, increased dryness, or loss of curl pattern, and adjust styling routines as needed.

By adhering to these best practices, both professionals and clients can incorporate heat styling safely and sustainably, maintaining the beauty, strength, and versatility of highly textured hair over time.

## Chemical Threshold™

**Chemical Threshold™** refers to the hair's ability to tolerate chemical-induced structural alteration before the integrity of the fiber becomes compromised. Chemical services such as lightening, coloring, relaxing, texturizing, permanent waving, and smoothing systems intentionally shift the hair beyond its natural pH equilibrium in order to alter the strand's internal structure. As the cuticle swells and the cortex becomes more accessible, the hair's resistance, elasticity, porosity, and overall stability begin to influence how safely and predictably the service can be performed. Hair with High Resistance™ typically maintains stronger structural stability during processing and may require more controlled penetration strategies to achieve the desired result. Hair with Balanced Integrity™ demonstrates a more predictable response, maintaining elasticity and recoverability when processed appropriately. Hair with Compromised Integrity™, however, has reduced structural stability and increased vulnerability due to repeated stress, excessive processing, or cumulative threshold exceedance, resulting in rapid chemical penetration, weakened elasticity, and elevated breakage risk. Understanding Chemical Threshold™ allows professionals to evaluate not only whether a chemical service can be performed, but whether the hair currently possesses the structural integrity necessary to safely achieve the client's desired result. *View Threshold Diagnostic Tables - See Appendix.*

**High Resistance™**

Hair with High Resistance™ demonstrates a stronger ability to maintain structural stability during chemical services and typically resists rapid chemical penetration. This hair often requires more intentional formulation selection, saturation techniques, extended processing strategies, or controlled heat support to achieve the desired level of alteration. High Resistance™ hair may present with compact cuticle layers, lower porosity tendencies, resistant graying patterns, coarse strand diameters, or virgin texture states that slow penetration and processing speed. While this hair can often tolerate chemical services more effectively than compromised hair, resistance should never be mistaken for invincibility. Excessive force, unnecessary overlapping, or prolonged exposure can still push the hair beyond its threshold and compromise its integrity.

**Balanced Integrity™**

Hair with Balanced Integrity™ demonstrates a stable and predictable response to chemical processing while maintaining manageable elasticity, structural resilience, and recoverability. This range represents hair that can generally tolerate controlled chemical services without immediate structural destabilization when proper professional protocols are followed. Balanced Integrity™ hair often displays moderate porosity, stable elasticity retention, consistent lift or deposit behavior, and controlled swelling during processing. Because the structure remains relatively balanced, the hair is more likely to recover effectively with appropriate post-service care, conditioning, and maintenance. This threshold range is often considered the most ideal for achieving reliable chemical outcomes while preserving the long-term health and performance of the fiber.

**Compromised Integrity™**

Hair with Compromised Integrity™ has reduced structural stability and increased vulnerability due to repeated stress, excessive processing, cumulative threshold exceedance, or chronic environmental and mechanical damage. This hair often experiences rapid chemical penetration because the protective structure of the cuticle and cortex has already been weakened or destabilized. Signs may include high porosity, elasticity collapse, mushy or brittle texture response, excessive swelling, cuticle erosion, thinning ends, uneven processing behavior, or significant breakage risk. In this threshold range, the hair may no longer possess the structural strength necessary to safely tolerate aggressive chemical alteration. Professional decision-making should shift toward stabilization, restorative care, corrective strategies, and long-term integrity preservation rather than immediate transformation.

**pH Effect on Hair Structure and Hair Bonds**

**pH, or "Potential Hydrogen,"** measures how acidic or alkaline a substance is on a scale from 0 to 14. A pH below 7 is **Acidic**, 7 is **Neutral**, and anything above 7 is **Alkaline**. Healthy hair, scalp, and skin naturally function within a slightly acidic range of approximately 4.5 to 5.5. This slightly acidic environment helps keep the cuticle compact, smooth, and protective. When hair remains within this balanced range, it retains moisture more effectively, reflects light for increased shine, maintains elasticity, and experiences less frizz and breakage.

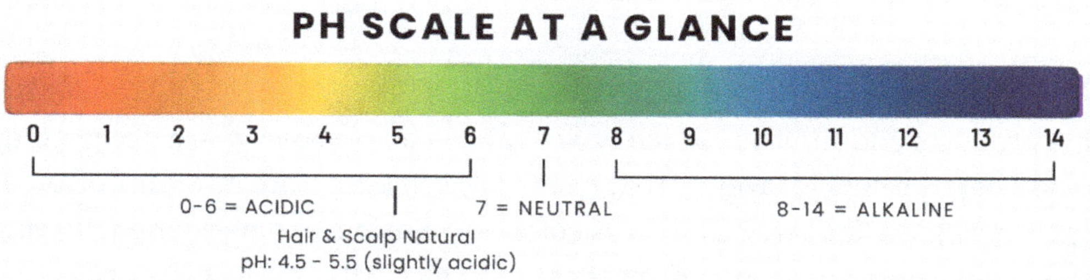


The pH of hair plays a critical role in the health, strength, appearance, and chemical behavior of the hair fiber. Almost every professional hair service involves a chemical reaction that alters the hair's structure by breaking, reshaping, or reforming internal bonds within the cortex. Services such as shampoos, relaxers, lighteners, hair color, and texturizers are not simply surface-level treatments. Even water can directly impact Hydrogen Bonds, while relaxers impact the structure of the hair, particularly the Disulfide Bonds that help give the hair its strength and form. Understanding pH allows professionals to predict how hair will respond during these services and make safer, more intentional decisions *See Chapter 2 Hair Structure*

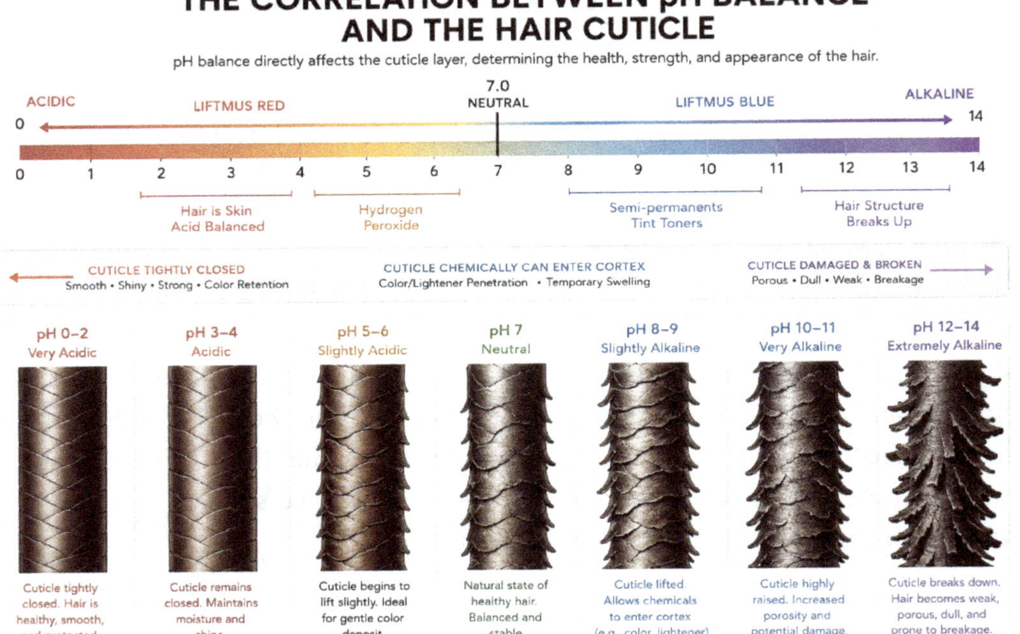


Alkaline products and services, which typically have a pH above 7, are designed to raise and open the cuticle layer so that chemicals can penetrate into the cortex. This process is necessary for services such as coloring, relaxing, and permanent waving. However, prolonged or uncontrolled exposure to high pH can cause excessive swelling of the hair shaft, increased porosity, moisture loss, dryness, brittleness, frizz, color fading, and structural weakness. Because the cuticle remains lifted, the hair becomes more vulnerable to damage and breakage if proper corrective steps are not taken afterward.

Acidic products, on the other hand, help restore and maintain the integrity of the hair. Slightly acidic formulas smooth and tighten the cuticle, helping the hair retain moisture, improve elasticity, reduce frizz, and preserve color longevity. Conditioners, bond treatments, and shine treatments commonly function within this lower pH range to rebalance the hair after chemical processing. These products support the hair's protective barrier and help restore strength and manageability.

**pH Control Journey**

Professional hair services should be viewed as a controlled pH journey. The process often begins by intentionally raising the pH to open the cuticle and allow the service

1
OPEN THE CUTICLE (IF NEEDED)
Raise pH (Alkaline)
Alkaline products lift the cuticle to allow access into the cortex.
• Cuticle opens
• Allows chemical penetration
• Risk of moisture loss & damage increases
pH 8–14
ALKALINE
2
PERFORM THE SERVICE
Chemical Action Occurs
The product works inside the cortex to achieve the desired result.
• Bonds are broken or restructured
• Hair changes shape or color
• Timing & strength must be controlled
CONTROL + MONITOR
3
RESTORE THE CUTICLE
Lower pH (Acidic)
Acidic products close and smooth the cuticle, restoring balance and protection.
• Cuticle closes
• Locks in moisture
• Reduces porosity
• Restores strength and shine
pH 0–6
ACIDIC

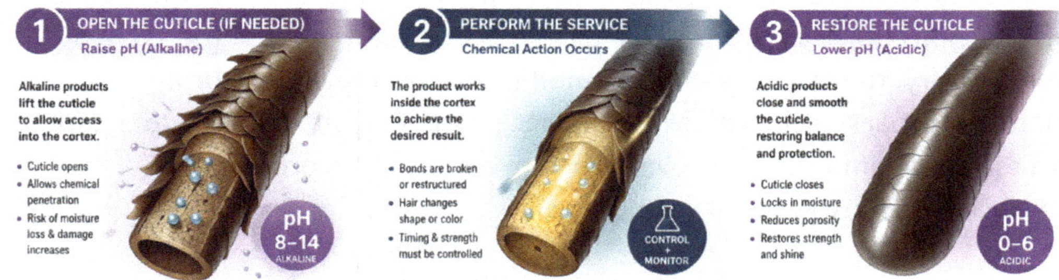

to work inside the cortex. Once the desired chemical action has occurred, the hair must then be guided back down into a slightly acidic state to close and smooth the cuticle. This final restoration step is essential for reducing porosity, locking in moisture, supporting strength, and stabilizing the final result. When this step is skipped or poorly executed, the cuticle can remain open, leaving the hair compromised, unpredictable, fragile, and difficult to manage.

**Overexposure** occurs when the hair or scalp is processed beyond its tolerance level. Signs of overexposure may include excessive softness, mushiness, abnormal stretching without recovery, breakage, irritation, redness, tingling, or burning

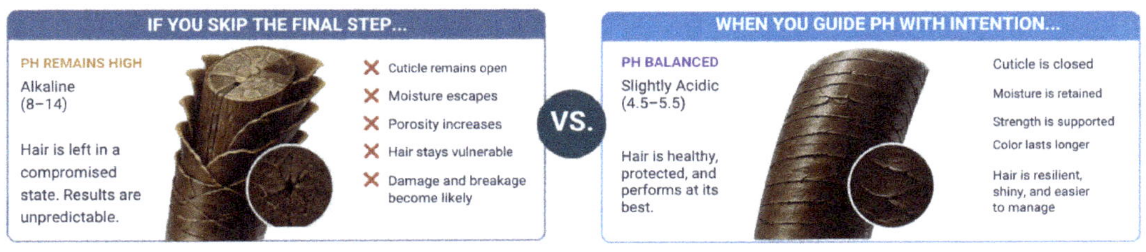

sensations. These are warning signs that the hair or scalp is becoming damaged. Rather than relying on guesswork, professionals should understand how to intentionally control pH, predict outcomes, and protect the integrity of both the hair and scalp throughout the service.

**Chemical burns** are injuries caused by excessive chemical exposure to the skin or scalp, and should not be considered a normal part of hair services. Certain areas, such as the edges, nape, and previously irritated scalp regions, are especially vulnerable because they are more delicate and prone to irritation or incomplete rinsing. Because of this, proper consultation and scalp analysis are critical before every chemical service. Professionals should assess for sensitivity, inflammation, lesions, previous reactions, or contraindications that may increase the client's risk. When necessary, the service should be modified, vulnerable areas protected, alternative approaches chosen, or the service postponed altogether. Protecting the client's scalp, hair integrity, and overall safety is part of the professional responsibility of every licensed cosmetologist.

## Mechanical Stress™

**Mechanical Stress™** encompasses all types of physical forces applied to the hair and scalp, ranging from common daily grooming to extreme practices that can greatly affect hair health when performed without consideration of the hair's elasticity, porosity, density, texture, and history of damage or chemical exposure. Mechanical Stress impacts the hair's Manipulation Threshold, Tension Threshold, and Friction Threshold. Several examples of mechanical stress that greatly affect hair health, include:

- **Excessive Styling Tool Use:** Aggressive or excessive brushing, combing, and detangling can cause fractures in the hair cuticle and damage to the scalp. Wet hair is particularly vulnerable, as it is more elastic and prone to stretching beyond its capacity. Using brushes with harsh bristles or fine-toothed combs can exacerbate this issue, especially when detangling knots.
- **Repetitive Styling**: Consistently styling hair in the same way over an extended period can gradually result in structural damage, mainly due to the continual

mechanical stress applied to specific areas. Hairstyles such as tight ponytails, braids, buns, and hair extensions can exert constant stress on the scalp and hair shaft. Over time, this weakens the structural bonds and heightens the risk of breakage.

- **Repetitive Sectioning**: Consistently sectioning the hair in the same pattern for treatments or styling can lead to variations in the hair structure across different sections. This occurs because certain areas may be over or under-exposed to product application or stressors. As a result, these sections of hair may become more prone to excessive porosity, dryness, or thinning compared to others.
- **Permanent Parts**: Consistently parting the hair in the same area (e.g., middle or side part) exposes certain areas of the scalp to repeated environmental and styling stressors. Over time, this can lead to thinning of the hairline or visibly sparse areas along the part line.
- **Excessive Layering of Products**: Continuously layering products like leave-ins, stylers, oils, or gels without proper cleansing leads to product buildup, which suffocates the strand and scalp. This not only dulls hair but also encourages scalp congestion, irritation, and flaking.
- **Excessive Use of Hair Accessories**: Certain hair accessories, like bands, clips, or hairpins, can introduce stress to the hair shaft. These accessories can snag or break hair strands, especially if used repeatedly in the same areas. Opting for gentler alternatives, such as fabric-covered elastics or scrunchies, can help mitigate this risk.
- **Backcombing (Teasing):** Backcombing involves combing hair against its natural direction to create volume. This technique can lift the cuticle layer, leading to increased porosity and vulnerability to damage. Regular backcombing can weaken hair over time, making it more susceptible to breakage. Offer suggestions to provide more clarity and professional soundness. Also, provide indicators that the manipulation threshold has been passed, and ways to mitigate damage caused by passing the manipulation threshold.

# Manipulation Threshold™

**Manipulation Threshold** refers to the maximum mechanical stress and product application that the hair and follicles can endure before experiencing structural compromise, such as cuticle damage, breakage, or excessive shedding. Understanding this threshold is essential for preserving hair integrity, particularly in textured, chemically treated, or naturally fragile hair types. When the Manipulation Threshold is exceeded, the cuticle layer becomes compromised, leading to dryness, increased frizz, tangling, brittleness, and eventual breakage. Repetitive strain may also affect the hair follicle, potentially resulting in scalp sensitivity, excessive shedding, or long-term thinning. *View Mechanical Threshold Diagnostic Tables - See Appendix.*

Indicators that the Manipulation Threshold has been exceeded can be present in several noticeable ways. One of the most common signs is the presence of short, snapped strands, which differ from normal shedding that releases full-length hairs from the follicle. Another key indicator is a loss of elasticity, where the hair stretches under tension but fails to return to its original shape or snaps easily. Hair may also exhibit excessive frizz and persistent tangling, becoming difficult to manage even with proper product use. A dry, brittle texture, particularly after conditioning, signals that the cuticle may be compromised and the strand is lacking moisture retention. Over time, you may observe thinning areas, especially along the hairline, parts, or nape, where repeated tension or styling practices are often concentrated. Additionally, the scalp may become tender, inflamed, or increasingly sensitive, especially in areas receiving the most manipulation. Finally, the appearance of various forms of strand damage further confirms that the hair's structural threshold has been breached.

## Types of Hair Strand Damage

Understanding the various types of hair strand damage is essential to maintaining healthy, resilient hair. Each form of damage presents distinct characteristics, causes, and approaches for prevention and repair. One of the most recognizable forms of damage is the **Split End**, where the hair strand divides at the tip in a "Y" shape. This typically results from dryness, friction, heat styling, or neglecting regular trims. Prevention involves trimming the ends regularly to remove weakened fibers, while smoothing serums or conditioners can temporarily bind and protect frayed ends from further splitting.

A more discreet form of damage is the **Needle-Eye Split**, which appears as a small, isolated slit anywhere along the hair shaft, resembling the eye of a needle. These are often caused by friction from brushing or abrasive, aggressive styling techniques, and overall hair dryness. They may also indicate deeper health concerns or nutritional deficiencies. Addressing this type of damage involves consistent moisturizing, reducing friction with satin or silk accessories, and gentle detangling practices.

**Branched Splits** develop when a needle-eye split worsens and begins to unravel, forming a slivered or tapered shortened end to the strand, often resembling a tree branch. This indicates exposure of multiple cuticle layers and cortex damage, frequently caused by repeated mechanical stress or prolonged dryness. Deep conditioning and protein treatments help reinforce the hair structure, while avoiding rough brushing on dry strands prevents further deterioration.

Another serious form of damage is **Fractured Cuticles**, which present as small, bare sections on the strand where the cuticle layer has been stripped away. This leaves the internal structure vulnerable. Such damage typically stems from excessive heat styling, chemical processing, or poor moisture balance. To address this, apply treatments containing hydrolyzed proteins to temporarily fill gaps in the cuticle and limit the use of high heat or strong chemicals in styling.

**Excessive Shedding** goes beyond the normal daily loss of 50–100 strands. When shedding becomes noticeable through thinning or clumps of hair, it may be tied to hormonal shifts (such as during pregnancy, postpartum, or menopause), medical conditions like thyroid imbalances or hypertension, and external stressors. Nutritional deficiencies, particularly in iron, protein, and biotin, also play a role. Effective resolutions include addressing underlying health issues with medical guidance, ensuring a nutrient-rich diet, managing stress levels, and improving overall lifestyle habits, including adequate hydration and sleep.

Lastly, **Single-strand Knots**, also known as fairy knots, are tiny knots formed by tangles in individual strands, most commonly in curly and coily textures. These knots form when strands loop and knot around themselves, particularly during washing or detangling. Preventing knots involves minimizing shrinkage, keeping hair well-moisturized, sealing ends with oils, and using detangling brushes or wide-tooth combs to manage the hair gently, especially when wet.

Several broader factors affect overall hair strand health. Hormonal fluctuations, such as those experienced during pregnancy or menopause, can influence the hair growth cycle. Medical conditions like thyroid disorders, high blood pressure, or those requiring chemotherapy can impair both the strength and growth of hair. Nutritional health is foundational, hair requires proteins, iron, and vitamins like biotin and vitamin D for strength and resilience. Adequate hydration is essential for maintaining scalp health and hair elasticity. Stress is another major disruptor, capable of triggering hair thinning or excessive shedding through hormonal imbalances. Finally, understanding your personal hair manipulation threshold, how much heat, tension, and product your hair can tolerate, helps avoid over-processing or mechanical damage.

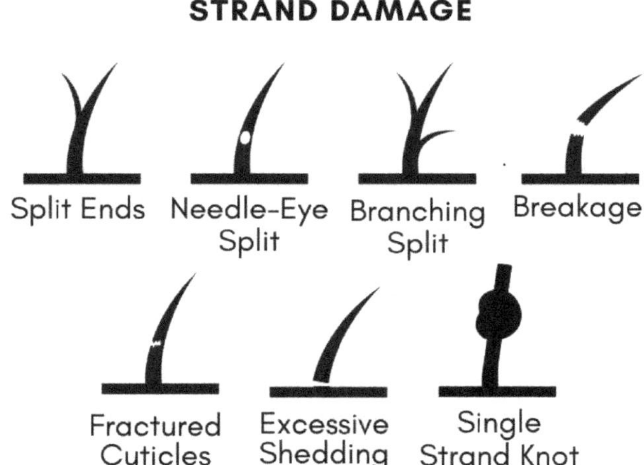


By recognizing these signs of damage and the contributing internal and external factors, professionals and clients alike can tailor hair care routines that protect and

individual's Tension Threshold must be considered, and the extensions must be worn strategically, sparingly, and with intentional breaks built into the cycle to truly preserve the integrity of both scalp and strands. Without this balance, what begins as a beauty enhancer can quietly become a root cause of long-term damage.

## Locs

The concept of Tension Threshold is just as relevant for individuals who wear locs over an extended period of time, but is often overlooked. Although locs are generally considered a low-manipulation style, they naturally accumulate weight over time. This weight isn't just from the locs themselves growing longer and thicker, but also from the accumulation of shed hair that would typically fall away in loose styles; this shed hair becomes compacted and held within the loc structure, contributing to a gradual increase in density and heaviness. As this weight builds, it begins to challenge the hair's Tension Threshold, especially at vulnerable areas like the crown and perimeter, which tend to have finer or less dense hair. Root tightening to maintain the locs as they grow can also be a great contributor to the weakening and damaging of the hair.

Over time, the constant downward pull of locs can lead to strain on the follicles, especially in the areas that bear the brunt of the heaviness, like the edges, nape, and crown. When the hair's natural tension threshold is exceeded consistently, follicular damage can occur, resulting in thinning, weakened roots, and even permanent hair loss in extreme cases. The issue is often subtle at first, with symptoms like scalp tenderness, widened parts, or thinning edges, but can become more pronounced over the years. In mature or long locs, gravity plays a role, as the weight tugs continuously on the scalp. To mitigate this damage, maintenance practices, such as regular scalp stimulation or strategic trims to reduce loc weight, are necessary; otherwise, this beautiful and culturally rich tradition can unintentionally contribute to long-term tension-related damage.

It's important for long-term loc wearers to monitor changes in hair density, especially in the top of the head and perimeters, and to recognize that locs, while protective in nature, are not immune to the effects of stress and weight. Respecting the hair's tension threshold through mindful care and restorative breaks is essential for sustaining both scalp health and loc longevity.

# Friction Thresholds™

**Friction Threshold** refers to the hair's ability to withstand repeated physical interaction with materials such as fabrics, styling tools, accessories, extensions, and wigs, without experiencing damage. When the Friction Threshold is exceeded, the hair becomes vulnerable to strand damage, frizzing, tangling, breakage, and moisture loss. This threshold is particularly important for highly textured hair, which often has a raised cuticle layer that makes it more susceptible to abrasion. Friction can come from a variety of sources, including cotton pillowcases, wool hats, synthetic scarves, tight braids, wig caps, and extensions. *View Mechanical Threshold Diagnostic Tables - See Appendix.*

Friction primarily impacts the cuticle layer of the hair strand. When the cuticle is repeatedly disturbed, it begins to lift or erode, leading to increased porosity, roughness, and an inability to retain moisture. This, in turn, affects elasticity and strength, weakening the hair over time and leading to mid-shaft breakage, split ends, a dull, frizzy appearance, and compromised texture shape. Friction can also thin out high-contact areas along the scalp, like the hairline, nape, or crown, especially when caused by tight wigs, ill-fitting extensions, or accessories like elastic headbands and rough headwraps.

To assess the friction threshold, professionals should analyze areas of the hair and scalp that may begin to appear compromised and find what repeated practices the client has begun. Ask the client how the hair reacts after a day of wearing scarves, hats, or wigs, and if there are signs of dryness or tangling that may suggest friction sensitivity. It's also important to note how hair responds to specific styles or accessories, especially if certain areas show signs of chronic damage.

Some styles and materials generate high friction and should be approached with caution, especially for clients with fragile or low-friction-threshold hair. These include tight box braids made with rough synthetic fibers, cornrows under wigs that are installed too tightly, crochet braids, lace wigs glued directly to the edges, nylon or cotton wig caps, and hats or scarves with rough linings. Daily-wear items such as tight elastic headbands or ponytail holders, and even frequently worn headwraps, can also cause damage if used too often without proper moisture and protection.

To help safeguard the hair, professionals should recommend using satin or silk-lined fabrics for pillowcases, bonnets, scarves, and wig caps. Encourage the client to limit the amount of time the hair is restricted and experiences friction. Moisturizing the hair before applying friction-heavy styles is essential, as hydrated hair resists damage more effectively. Barrier products like lightweight oils or leave-in conditioners can reduce direct contact and soften the impact of friction. Additionally, clients should be encouraged to alternate styles, rest the hair between protective looks, and choose high-quality, smooth extensions that are less abrasive. Wigs should be properly fitted to avoid movement that leads to scalp rubbing, and satin wig grips can be used to minimize friction.

Exceeding the friction threshold doesn't always lead to immediate, obvious damage. It tends to erode the hair slowly. However, over time, chronic friction can compromise the hair's structural integrity, particularly when combined with other stressors like heat, manipulation, and tension. This can result in long-term thinning, loss of length, difficulty retaining moisture, and overall decline in hair health. Recognizing and respecting the friction threshold allows stylists and clients alike to preserve the hair's natural strength, appearance, and resilience.

## Texture Recovery™

**Texture Recovery™** is the hair's response to external stress or a change in internal conditions, assessed by whether the hair returns to, adapts from, or is unable to reestablish its natural Texture Shape and Texture Pattern. After every service, whether thermal styling, chemical processing, or mechanical stress, you should assess the hair to see what it has experienced. Does it return to its original Texture Shape? Does it hold a new Texture Pattern? Or does it struggle with incongruency, unable to find any consistent shape or pattern at all?

What is visible on the outside is always a reflection of what has taken place within the strand. At the structural level, the hair responds to stress in one of three ways:

- Bonds may shift temporarily, allowing the hair to return to its original shape
- Bonds may reset into a new configuration, resulting in a lasting change in shape without compromising overall integrity

- Bonds may break or degrade, leading to inconsistency, weakness, and loss of pattern.

**The Three Outcomes of Texture Recovery**

**Recovered Texture™** is the outcome in which the hair fully returns to its **Natural State™,** maintaining its unaltered Texture Shape and Texture Pattern. The strands behave as they did prior to the intervention, indicating that the thresholds were respected and the hair's internal structure remains intact.

**Altered Hair™** is the outcome in which the hair does not return to its Natural State™, specifically its original Texture Shape or Pattern. Within the structure of Texture Recovery, the hair maintains its structural integrity but exists in an **Altered State™** due to an intervention. In an Altered State, one or more thresholds are exceeded, resetting the hair's shape while preserving its internal structure. As a result, the hair adapts to a new, consistent configuration. This is not damage. The strands may appear looser, elongated, or even straight, yet they remain healthy, flexible, and resilient. This outcome is most commonly observed in cases of heat training.

**Compromised Texture™** is the outcome in which the hair loses its ability to maintain a consistent or recognizable pattern due to structural disruption from exceeded thresholds. This leaves the hair in a **Damaged State™**, a condition in which structural integrity has been disrupted due to threshold exceedance, resulting in fragility, inconsistency, and a loss of functional integrity. The hair may feel weak, overly soft, brittle, or prone to breakage. This occurs when one or more thresholds are exceeded, beyond the hair's structural tolerance. The hair may need to be cut or trimmed to remove the damage.

**A Critical Distinctions: Altered vs. Compromised, Texture Recovery vs. Texture State**

One of the most common misunderstandings in highly textured hair care is the assumption that any failure to return to the natural pattern indicates damage. This is not always true. Unlike Texture Compromised hair, Texture Altered hair retains its integrity and may gradually return toward its original pattern over time, or it may maintain its new configuration permanently; both can maintain a healthy structure.

Texture Recovery is not a standing classification. The outcome of this assessment may inform or update the hair's Texture State, but the two frameworks serve different evaluative purposes. Texture State answers the question, *"Where is this hair right now in its overall journey?"* It is a snapshot of the hair's relationship to its original structure at any given point in time. Texture Recovery answers the question, *"How did this hair respond to what I just did to it?"* It is an assessment of the reaction, evaluated in the context of a specific service. It is a post-service diagnostic, not a standing classification.

A lack of Texture Recovery does not automatically indicate compromised integrity. Understanding this distinction allows for more accurate assessment, more appropriate treatment decisions, and more informed communication with clients. This line of thinking shifts the approach from assumption to analysis. It allows the professional to respond with intention rather than reaction.

## Key Terms

**Hair Thresholds™**: The tolerance limit that hair has for various external stressors and internal deficiencies.

**Protein Threshold™**: The maximum amount of protein your hair can absorb before it starts to experience adverse effects.

**Protein State™**: The protein levels in the hair at any given time.

**Protein Overload™**: When hair exceeds its protein threshold.

**Moisture Threshold™**: The maximum level of hydration or moisture loss that hair can absorb without compromising its structural integrity.

**Hydration**: The act of increasing the hair's water content.

**Moisturization™**: The process of sealing and protecting hydration by forming a barrier around the hair strand.

**Sealants™**: Hydrophobic (water-repelling) substances that create a protective barrier over the hair shaft.

**Moisture Level™**: The amount of water content within the hair strands.

**Hygral Fatigue**: Weakening of the hair as it undergoes repeated swelling and contracting due to excessive moisture.

**Moisture Cycle™**: The natural process in which hair absorbs, retains, and loses moisture over time.

**Moisture Retention Regimen™**: A routine of layering hydrators and moisturizers to maintain a healthy moisture level.

**Heat Threshold™**: The point at which hair can no longer endure thermal exposure without experiencing structural changes.

**Heat Response™**: how the hair responds to exposure to heat

**Unaltered Response™**: The state of hair in which there is no permanent change to the hair's structure from thermal exposure, and it easily reverts to its original natural texture shape without lasting effects.

**Heat Training™**: The controlled use of moderate heat over time to loosen the natural texture.

**Heat Damage™**: The result of when hair's heat threshold is exceeded.

**Heat Delivery™**: How heat is administered to hair during a service.

**Atmospheric Heat™**: A distribution of heat into the atmosphere surrounding the hair.

**Direct Heat™**: The immediate transfer of heat from the heat source to the hair's surface.

**Steam Heat™**: A heat distribution that introduces warmth alongside water vapor, allowing the hair to expand rather than contract.

**Radiant Heat™**: A distribution of infrared heat that increases penetration by warming the hair from within.

**Ionic Influenced Heat™**: A heat distribution that involves applying heat while releasing negative ions to break water molecules into smaller particles.

**Chemical Threshold™**: The hair's ability to tolerate chemical-induced structural alteration before the integrity of the fiber becomes compromised. Chemical

**High Resistance™:** Hair that demonstrates a stronger ability to maintain structural stability during chemical services and typically resists rapid chemical penetration.

**Manipulation Threshold™**: The maximum mechanical stress and product application that the hair and follicles can endure.

**Balanced Integrity™:** Hair that demonstrates a stable and predictable response to chemical processing while maintaining manageable elasticity, structural resilience, and recoverability.

**Compromised Integrity™:** Hair that has reduced structural stability and increased vulnerability due to repeated stress, excessive processing, cumulative threshold exceedance, or chronic environmental and mechanical damage.

**pH, or "Potential Hydrogen":** How acidic or alkaline a substance is on a scale from 0 to 14.

**Acidic:** A pH below 7

**Neutral:** A pH of

**Alkaline:** A pH above 7

**Overexposure:** When the hair or scalp is subjected to a chemical process beyond its tolerance level.

**Chemical burns**: Injuries caused by excessive chemical exposure to the skin or scalp

**Mechanical Stress™**: All types of physical forces applied to the hair and scalp.

**Split End**: The hair strand divides at the tip in a "Y" shape.

**Needle-Eye Split**: A small, isolated slit anywhere along the hair shaft.

**Branched Splits™**: A slivered or tapered shortened strand end resembling a tree branch.

**Fractured Cuticles™**: A small, bare section on the strand where the cuticle layer has been stripped away.

**Excessive Shedding™**: Hair shedding that goes beyond the normal daily loss of 50–100 strands.

**Single-Strand Knots**: Tiny knots formed by tangles in individual strands.

**Tension Threshold™**: The point at which a hair fiber can be stretched or elongated without compromising its structural integrity.

**Friction Threshold™**: The hair's ability to withstand repeated physical interaction with materials.

**Texture Recovery™**: The hair's response to a service, assessed by whether the hair returns to, adapts from, or is unable to reestablish its natural Texture Movement™.

**Recovered Texture™**: The Texture Recovery outcome in which the hair fully returns to its Natural State™.

**Natural State™™:** The condition of hair that retains its original structure, Texture Shape™, and Texture Pattern™ without permanent deviation.

**Altered State™**: The state in which one or more thresholds are exceeded, resetting the hair's shape while preserving its internal structure.

**Compromised Texture™**: The Texture Recovery outcome in which the hair loses its ability to maintain a consistent or recognizable pattern due to structural disruption from exceeded thresholds.

**Damaged State™**: The condition of hair in which structural integrity has been disrupted due to threshold exceedance, resulting in incongruent texture, weakness, brittleness, or loss of pattern

# 6. Scalp Spatial Distribution ™

*Service Customization Through Mapping Trait-Based Scalp Commonalities*

The scalp is made up of key anatomical and styling reference points that guide salon services, from cutting and coloring to updos, braids, locs, and extensions. Among the most referenced are the **Front Corners** of the front hairline, which mark the transition from the center of the hairline to the temples. The Front Corners are often where baby hairs or signs of recession appear. The **Apex**, the highest point of the head, is essential for balancing parts, sections, and volume. Just behind it, the **Crown** that tends to be a dense area of hair, prone to growth whorls and puffiness. The **Parietal Ridge**, curving above the ears, helps shape silhouettes and guide blend lines. The **Temples**, between the corners of the hairline and the top of the ear, are typically sparse and sensitive to tension. **Sideburns**, present in all genders, extend from the temple to the jawline and vary in density. The **Occipital region**, centered at the back of the head, supports weight and serves as a critical anchoring zone. Below it, the **Nape** transitions to the neck with finer, downward-growing, low-density hair. The **Mastoid Process**, a bony point just behind the ear, is often used to maintain balance and alignment when shaping, coloring, braiding, or installing extensions.

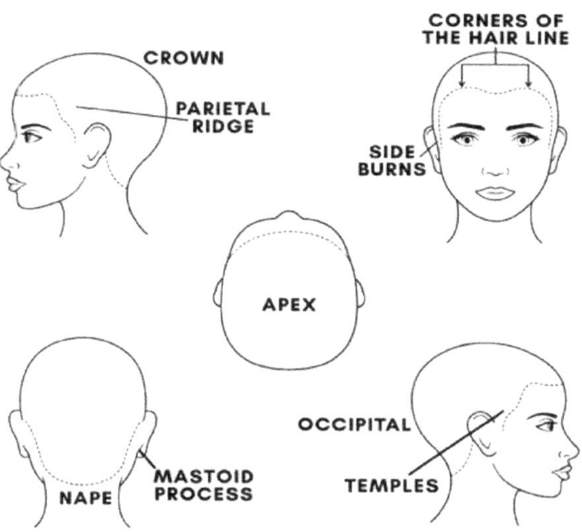

# Scalp Spatial Distribution

**Scalp Spatial Distribution (SSD)** is a trait-based scalp mapping method that enables stylists to deliver customized, precision-based hair care. SSD encourages professionals to evaluate the scalp across 3 anchors and 12 distinct zones, each defined by bone structure and the commonality of hair traits found in that region. These regions include:

- **Front Hair Line:** The edge of the scalp above the forehead, spanning from temple to temple.
- **Back Hair Line:** The lower boundary of the scalp at the nape, extending from behind one ear to the other.
- **Central Line:** The midline of the scalp running from the front hairline to the back hairline.
- **Corners of the Hair Line**: The left and right points of the front hairline, between the central line and the temple zone, where the hairline changes direction, and the outermost points where the back hairline meets the nape boundary, functioning as reference markers that establish balance, guide sectioning, and align placement across styling, cutting, and coloring services.
- **Left Side:** The section between the central line and the left ear, from the front to the back hairline.
- **Right Side:** The section between the central line and the right ear, from the front to the back hairline.
- **Front Perimeter:** The border zone framing the forehead and temple area, from in front of the ear to the other ear.
- **Temple:** The area between the end of the eyebrows and the top of the ears, forward of the parietal ridge.
- **Front:** The area spanning from ear to ear, over the apex, and forward to the front hairline.
- **U Section:** A U-shaped area from the front corners of the hairline, extending back to the crown.
- **Top:** The area from the occipital forward to the front perimeter, between the parietal ridges.
- **Crown:** The region behind the apex and above the occipital.

- **Back:** The area spanning from ear to ear, over the apex, and down to the back hairline.
- **Occipital Band™:** The horizontal band beneath the crown and above the nape, extending from behind one ear to the other.
- **Nape:** The lowest portion of the scalp, just beneath the occipital bone, extending to the top of the neck.
- **Back Perimeter:** The lower edge of the scalp, from ear to ear across the nape, down to the hairline.

By analyzing the scalp as a mapped system of functional regions, stylists can better anticipate hair behavior, customize techniques, reinforce weak and fragile areas, and create services that are not only visually balanced but technically sound and long-lasting. The following section provides a breakdown of these 15 areas and the traits most commonly found within each area.

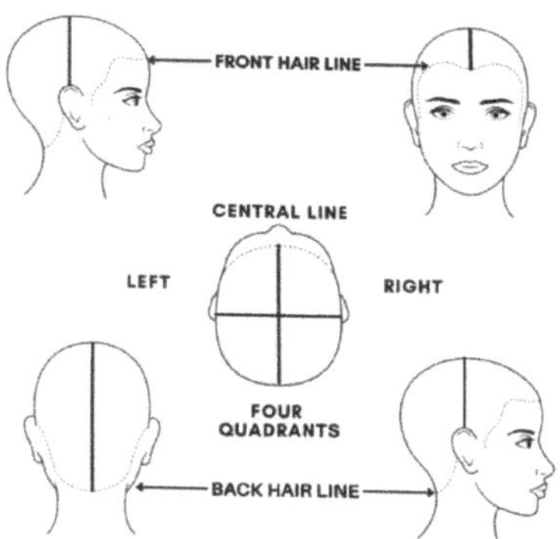


The first three areas of the SSD are the Front Hair Line, Back Hair Line, and Central Line. They are considered **Anchors™** on the scalp because they serve as natural dividing lines and reference markers that help define sectioning, balance, directionality, and are critical to styling symmetry and tension control. The **Front Hairline** is typically composed of finer, lower-density strands and is highly exposed to tension and environmental factors, making it more fragile and more likely to show signs of breakage or thinning. Similarly, the **Back Hairline**, the lowest area of the Nape, while slightly more resilient, tends to have a fine to medium texture and moderate density but is often affected by friction and tension-related dryness or breakage, contact with clothes, and in styles that anchor in this area. The **Central Line**, extending from the center point of the front hairline to the center point of the nape, commonly features growth swirls or cowlicks that define natural parting patterns and directional fall. This area is key in determining sectioning for styling and cutting, as well as the **Four Quadrants**, four sections divided down the center line and across from ear to ear, over the apex.

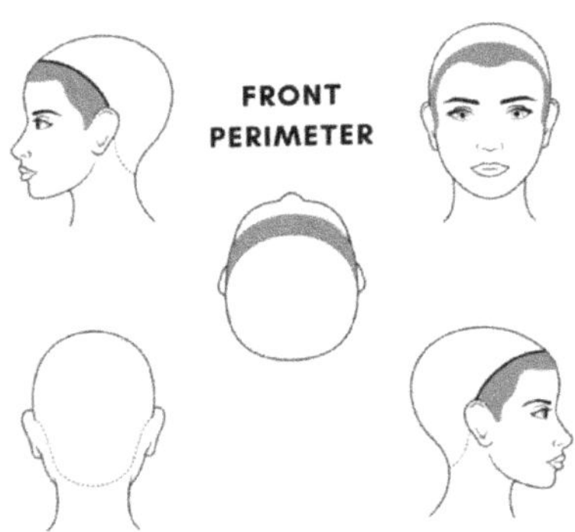


The **Front Perimeter** is a band running from parietal ridge to parietal ridge across the front of the head, framing the face. This area typically features moderate to fine Strand Diameter and baby hairs. This area is crucial for seamless blending of styles and layering, as it determines the forward fall and fringe of the hair.

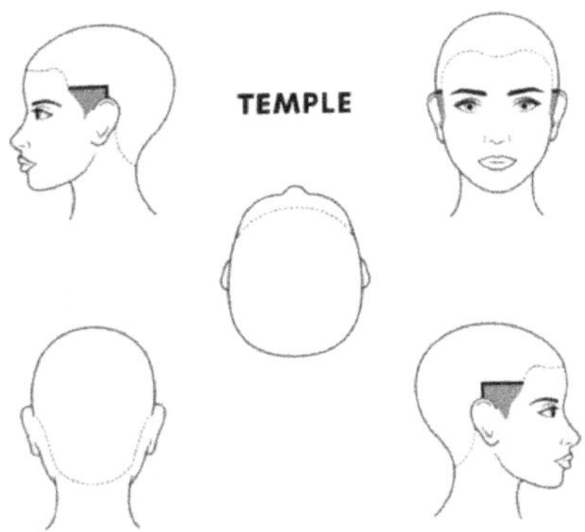


The lowest part of the Front Perimeter is the **Temple** area, located between the ear and front hairline. This area adds an incredible accent when styled in short cuts for both men and women. However, it can often be sparse and fragile, showing signs of breakage and thinning. Careful friction and tension management is needed in extension installations, styling, and even when wearing glasses.

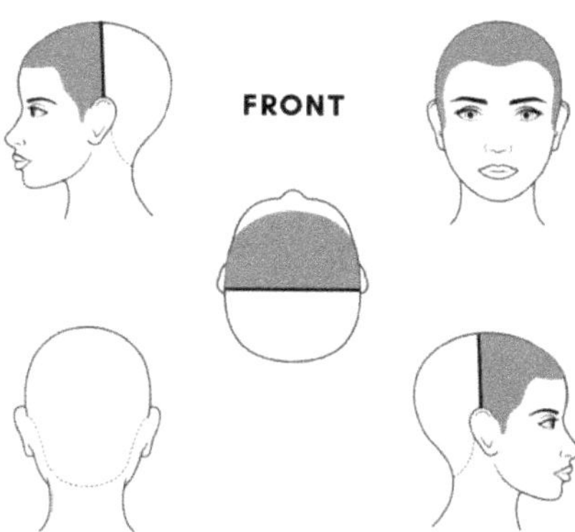


The **Front Of The Head**, from ear to ear over the apex forward to the hairline, combines multiple areas. The hair often tapers in density and Strand Diameter moving towards the hairline and the front corners of the front perimeter. This area often serves as an anchor for layered shapes and updos. Balance and symmetry are crucial in this area when installing braids, locs, and extensions.

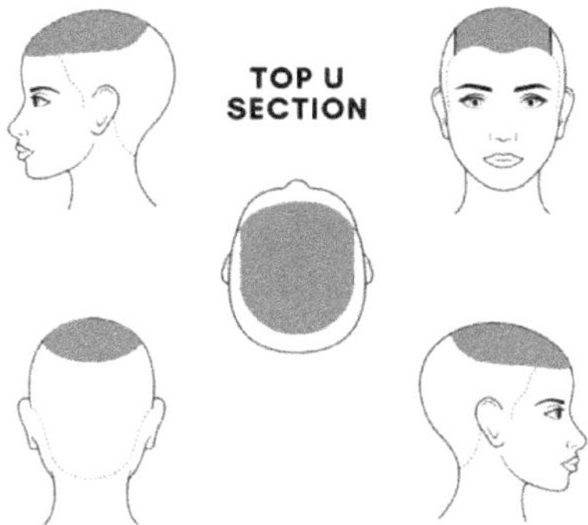


The **U Section** is a U-shaped region at the top of the head, parted at both eyebrow peaks backward, connecting above the crown. This area encompasses a combination of the crown and frontal hair characteristics. It is often softer in texture feel, less dense, and plays a pivotal role in style symmetry, layering, visual balance, movement, volume, and overall shape of the finished.

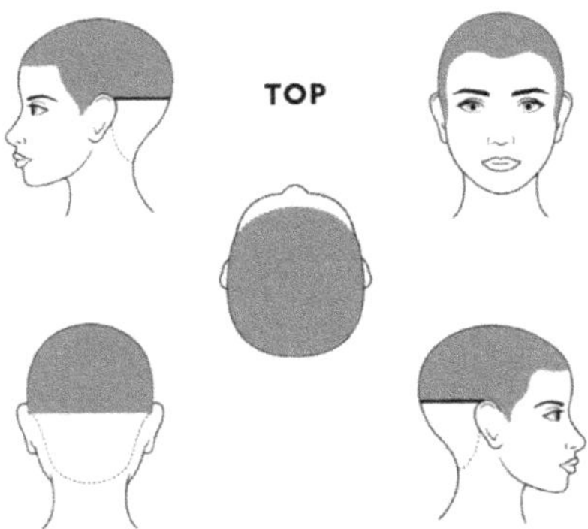


The **Top Of The Head**, from the occipital bone forward to the front perimeter, typically holds the majority of the hair and scalp surface. The area combines most scalp areas.

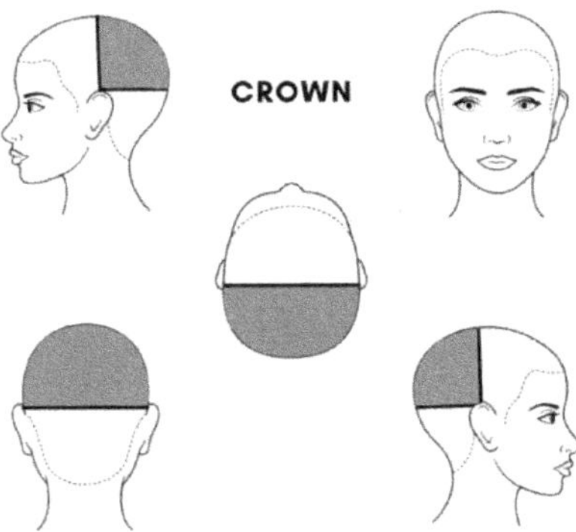


The **Crown**, located from ear to ear over the apex and back to the occipital region, is typically one of the densest areas of the scalp. It often contains strong follicular anchoring and retains significant heat. This makes it ideal for volume-building and critical when planning color and chemical service timing.

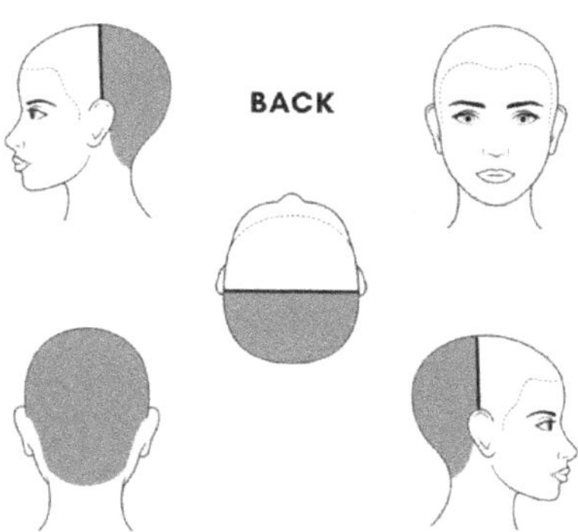


The **Back** region is the expansive area of the scalp that spans from one ear to the other, arches over the apex, and extends down to the back hairline. This region includes key sub-areas such as the crown, occipital, and nape, making it critical for managing volume, anchor support, and overall silhouette. Its curved structure influences how styles fall and hold in the back and plays a central role in cutting balance, extension installs, braiding layouts, and gradient color transitions.

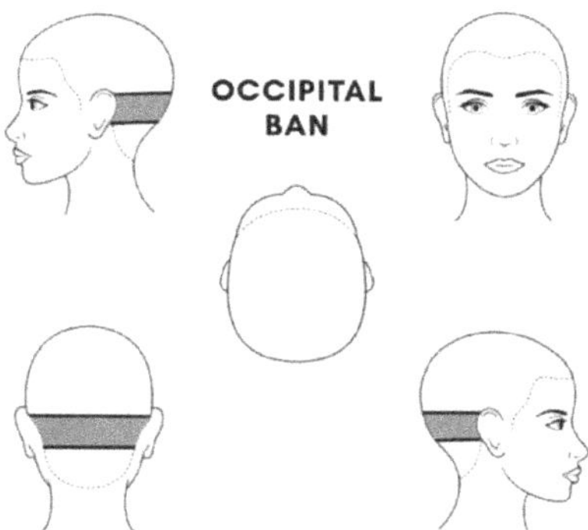


The **Occipital Band™**, from behind one ear, under the occipital bone, across to behind the other ear. This area is known for its high tension tolerance and is commonly used as an anchoring base for extensions, weaves, and braids, as it commonly has the highest hair density and thickest texture diameter, and scalp service space to consider when styling. This area can be the most resistant to chemical processing in shorter hair, while retaining more heat during chemical services for longer hair. This area also often has the most defined texture shape.

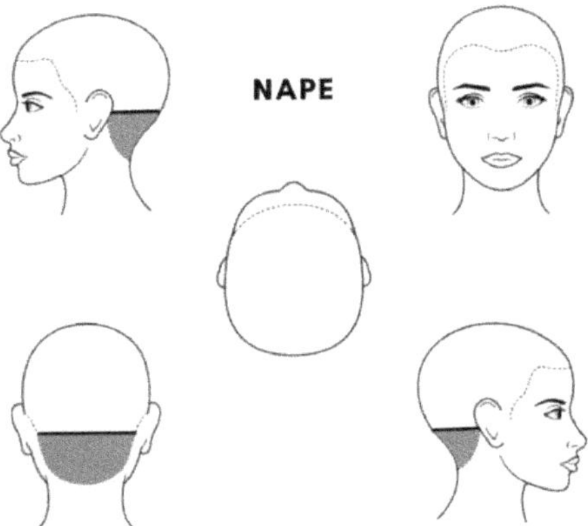


The **Nape**, extending from the occipital bone down to the back perimeter, has a downward growth direction and is often sensitive to tension. Its lower density and fragility make it a key area for breakage in high-manipulation styles.

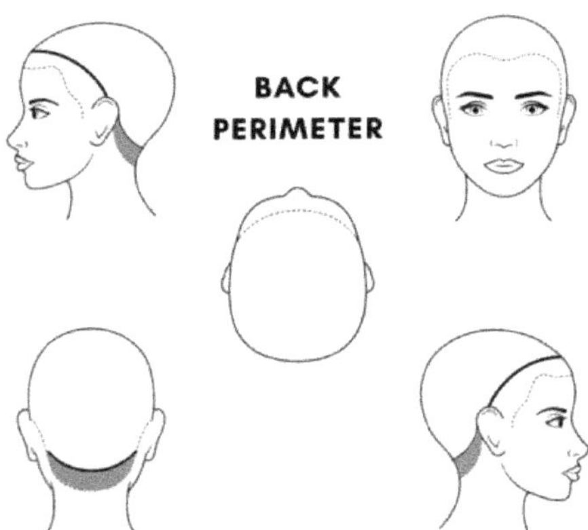


The **Back Perimeter** is ear to ear across the lower nape to the back hairline, and is an area that must be treated gently due to its typically fine texture and susceptibility to perimeter stress during styling or installations. This area also tends to have the tightest texture shape of all the areas of the head.

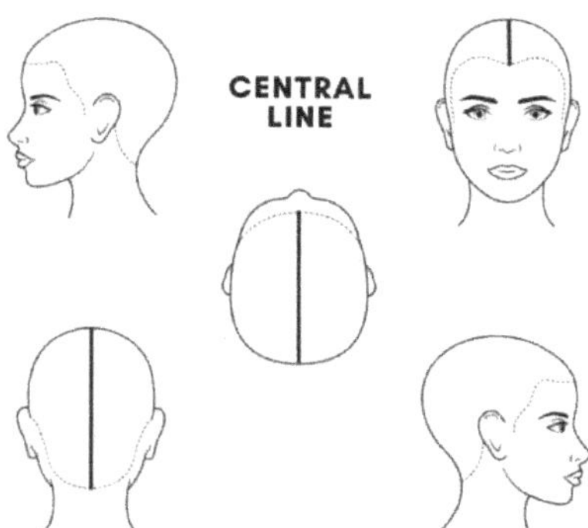


The **Left Side and Right Side**, defined as from the central line to the respective hairlines, often reveal slight differences in density and growth patterns due to natural asymmetry, sleeping positions, hand dominance, and repeated parting and sectioning. These side sections frequently require tailored adjustments in styling and cutting to ensure balance.

Regardless of the salon service, these defined areas work together to equip stylists with a roadmap to deliver precise, tailored, protective, and visually harmonious services. By observing the shared traits in each region, professionals can proactively plan and adjust techniques, sectioning, and product usage to optimize results and safeguard the client's hair health.

## The SSD Evaluation & Execution Framework™

The Scalp Spatial Distribution System™ is a system designed to build a fundamental foundation for understanding and working with hair textures. It is more than a technical reference; it embodies a mindset that influences salon professionalism, expertise, and customer relations by removing "One-size-fits-all" methodologies. Each scalp presents a unique landscape of texture, density, direction, and sensitivity, requiring distinct responses marked by precision, professionalism, and the preservation of the hair's long-term health. With this in mind, SSD is used to assess and plan strategy before the stylist picks up a styling tool, to ensure that they provide intentional, customized care, avoiding default routines. While it may not be realistic to apply every step with every client, this framework equips stylists with an expanded expertise, as well as language for training staff and communicating with customers.

To effectively utilize SSD mapping, stylists must follow a clear, repeatable process that transforms routine services into personalized, precision-based execution, using the SSD Evaluation & Execution Framework. The **SSD Evaluation & Execution Framework ™** is a methodology designed to guide stylists from consultation through to execution. In standard cosmetology instruction, consultations are conducted by analyzing four main hair properties: elasticity, texture, density, and porosity. Consider the SSD Framework to expand standard hair analysis to a step-by-step method for customizing hair services using Scalp Spatial Distribution. Understanding the scalp through SSD requires a basic awareness of how different areas of the head often share predictable hair traits. Each zone carries common characteristics that affect how hair responds to cutting, coloring, chemical treatments, styling, extension, loc, and braid installations.

- **Step 1 - Consultation**
  The process begins not with scissors or shampoo, but with a client-centered conversation. Stylists using the SSD method first engage in an in-depth discussion with their client to uncover their desired outcomes, hair history, sensitivities, and lifestyle factors. This foundation allows the stylist to contextualize what they see and feel during the analysis that follows. A client's gym routine, medical history, or previous color mishaps all provide valuable insight into how the hair and scalp may react during services, and how those services must be adapted.

- **Step 2 - Analysis of Hair Properties**
  Once the client's goals are clearly outlined, the first technical step of the SSD method is an observational analysis of hair traits across all scalp regions. Instead of only assessing the hair as a whole silhouette, the stylist does a deeper examination of each distinct region for hair characteristics that may vary throughout the head, i.e., elasticity, density, porosity, and strand diameter. This aids the stylist in anticipating how the hair behaves in varying ways, such as how it may respond in differing ways to heat, hold shape, accept product saturation, or create bulk in a finished cut. Recognizing these patterns early allows the stylist to anticipate challenges before they occur.

- **Step 3 - Analysis of Texture Indicators**
  After the foundational hair properties are identified across each zone, the stylist moves to the second step: analyzing the Texture Indicators of the client's

hair. This includes identifying Texture State (natural, altered, or transitioning), texture movement (texture shape, texture patterns, incongruency), strand diameter (fine, medium, coarse), and the feel of the texture (such as silky, cottony, or wiry). These textural signatures offer insights into how each region of the hair will behave during styling or chemical services. For instance, a cottony crown may puff up with moisture, while silky temples may struggle to hold volume or braid tension.

- **Step 4 – Threshold Check**
  With texture and hair property evaluations complete, the stylist now conducts a threshold check, the third key step in the SSD framework. This involves scanning each region of the scalp and hair for signs that it may have crossed or is approaching a critical stress point. These include the heat threshold (evidenced by altered texture shape, pattern, and elasticity), manipulation threshold (seen in excessive tangling or shedding), tension threshold (noted through hair thinning or scalp tenderness), friction threshold (manifesting as fraying or scalp irritation in areas like the nape or hairline), protein threshold (indicated by breakage or brittleness), and moisture threshold (seen in dryness or mushy elasticity). If any thresholds are compromised, the service plan must shift toward restoration and protection before aesthetic goals can be safely achieved.

- **Step 5 - SSD Service Plan™**
  Having thoroughly assessed the hair's characteristics, texture, behavior, and stress indicators, the stylist now enters the fourth step: designing a personalized SSD Service Plan. An **SSD Service Plan** is a diagrammed, customized, region-specific strategy for delivering hair services, guided by Scalp Spatial Distribution mapping. Using the observations collected, the stylist maps out each relevant scalp region and indicates the appropriate techniques, tools, and products needed to execute the desired service. This could mean using larger rods in denser regions of a rod set, reducing manipulation around fragile temples of a braid style, or adjusting the tension and placement of extensions in accordance with anchoring strength in the occipital band. This plan ensures that each region receives what it needs, not just what the style

requires. With time, a written diagram will not be necessary because a high level of technical expertise will be developed.

*Sample SSD Service Plan – See Appendix*

- **Step 6 - Client Communication**
  The sixth step in the framework is client communication. Here, the stylist takes time to walk the client through the plan, explaining what was observed, what will be done differently, and how that aligns with both the client's goal and the hair's current condition. This not only builds trust but also allows the client to become an active partner in the hair care journey, with realistic expectations and clear aftercare instructions.

- **Step 6 - Execution with SSD Awareness**
  Finally, the stylist moves into step seven, real-time execution with SSD awareness. As the service is carried out, the stylist stays engaged with the plan while remaining adaptable. Tension is adjusted based on how the scalp responds. Product quantity or placement may change if porosity reveals itself differently mid-service. The SSD-trained stylist works like a sculptor, making intelligent, nuanced adjustments as the hair communicates its needs zone by zone.

The SSD Evaluation & Execution Framework is not a checklist. It's a discipline, a mindset, and a method for elevating hair services into a practice of precision, efficiency, and customization. When stylists approach every head not as a canvas but as a map to be read and respected, they become stellar service providers. As stylists excel in training of the SSD Framework, they will be able to examine a head of hair and immediately see how to deconstruct and recreate any look a client references.

## Using SSD to Deconstruct Color Services

Scalp Spatial Distribution (SSD) offers a regionally guided, trait-based framework that elevates the way color services are planned and performed. Whether the goal is an all-over color, balayage, foils, or a more creative placement, SSD allows stylists to make thoughtful decisions based on how color behaves across different areas of the scalp, how the hair lies in its natural texture, and how scalp shape and density zones influence light reflection and visual balance. Rather than relying on uniform techniques, SSD encourages the stylist to evaluate where color should be applied for maximum dimension, how the head's shape affects highlight visibility, which regions may require adjusted saturation due to porosity or texture, and how light interacts with various parts of the head, both in natural fall and styled states. It also prompts an analysis of how curl or wave patterns affect the rhythm and perception of color transitions across the hair.

Color application is never one-size-fits-all. SSD reveals how the curvature of the scalp, differences in density, hair diameter, and styling preferences (natural vs. straightened texture) impact contrast, depth, and focal points. Each SSD region plays a specific role in how color is seen and felt within the finished design. For example, the crown and apex are natural focal points that catch light first. Because these zones can appear flat or overly dense depending on the texture shape, highlights in this area help elevate the cut with dimension, though stylists must be mindful of growth swirls that may cause uneven lift. The front hairline and temples, by contrast, are highly visible but fragile zones. These areas benefit from delicate, face-framing color like money pieces and baby-light foils. Due to their low density and fine texture, these regions require a gentle hand and controlled saturation.

The parietal ridge and sides serve as transitional bridges between the top and lower halves of the head. When building a color gradient, these zones help stylists determine where the intensity of highlights should shift. For straight styles, lightening may occur higher in this region, while for curly or coily styles, where shrinkage compresses visual length, color is often placed deeper within the ridge. The occipital and nape are typically denser, cooler-toned areas with more resistant porosity. These regions receive the least direct light, making them ideal for adding shadow, richness, or surprise contrast with peekaboo accents. The Top U-section is a dominant color zone where placement decisions define the brightness, softness, or contour of the entire look. Since this region is highly visible in both parted and free-flowing styles, SSD mapping ensures the brightness here is distributed harmoniously without overpowering the shape of the head.

SSD is also key in designing gradient balance and focal points throughout the hair. Using SSD mapping, stylists can plan brightness near the face, especially along the front corners, temples, and top front, while tapering off intensity toward the occipital or nape to preserve grounding and depth. In denser areas like the crown or back, stylists may use heavier saturation or thicker weaves, whereas finer regions like the temples benefit from soft, feathered strokes. Advanced color techniques like shadow rooting, zone toning, and drop foiling can all be guided by the natural topography of the scalp.

SSD can also influence the color planning for hair. Coily and curly hair may appear shorter due to shrinkage, compressing the visibility of lightened strands and requiring closer foil spacing or lower placement to preserve blend. When the hair is blown out or straightened, color placements may look bolder or more exaggerated. SSD supports stylists in anticipating these differences by ensuring they plan placement and contrast based on how the style will be worn, not just how it appears in the bowl or in foil. SSD ensures the result appears intentional and balanced, no matter how the client wears their hair, whether in curls, updos, or smooth, straight styles.

With SSD stylists assess how each zone contributes to the desired finish look and whether it should be enhanced, neutralized, deepened, or softened. Next, apply color theory to formulate appropriately, ensuring that regions with common traits are properly accounted for and volume.

## Integrating SSD with Color Theory for Customization and Dimension

Color theory begins with evaluating five essential elements: the client's current color level, their desired level, the underlying pigment exposed during lift, and their target color, including hue, level, and tone. Rather than applying these elements universally, SSD encourages stylists to analyze these factors per region to ensure full coverage, uniformity, consistency, balance, and desired dimension. For example, the frontal hairline and temples are typically finer and more porous, often lifting faster and requiring lower-volume developer or protective foil techniques. The crown and apex, however, are denser, making them more resistant to lift and prone to appearing flat without strategic brightness. The parietal ridge and sides involve curvature that affects light reflection and requires foil placement or balayage techniques that follow the contour of the head. The occipital and nape regions are denser and often contain more resistant pigment and may require stronger formulas or longer processing times to

## Key Words

**Front Corners:** The area of the front hairline, which mark the transition from the center of the hairline to the temples, which mark the transition from the center of the hairline to the temples.

**Apex**: The highest point of the head, located at the top-center of the head.

**Parietal Ridge**: The curved lateral section of the head that runs from the top of the ear upward toward the crown.

**Sideburns**: The vertical area that extends from the temple region down to the jawline, located in front of the ear.

**Occipital Region**: The rounded lower back portion of the skull, centered around the occipital bone.

**Mastoid Process**: A bony protrusion located just behind the earlobe.

**Scalp Spatial Distribution (SSD)™**: A trait-based method of mapping the scalp that enables stylists to deliver customized, precision-based hair care.

**Back Hair Line™**: The lower boundary of the scalp at the nape, extending from behind one ear to the other.

**Corners of the Hair Line™**: The left and right points of the front hairline, between the central line and the temple zone, where the hairline changes direction, and the outermost points where the back hairline meets the nape boundary.

**Temple**: The area between the end of the eyebrows and the top of the ears, forward of the parietal ridge.

**Front**: The area spanning from ear to ear, over the apex, and forward to the front hairline.

**Top™**: The area from the apex forward to the front perimeter, between the parietal ridges.

**Crown**: The upper back portion of the scalp, behind the apex and above the occipital.

**Anchors™**: The Front Hair Line, Back Hair Line, and Central Line that act as reference markers.

**Front Hair Line™**: The edge of the scalp above the forehead, spanning from temple to temple.

**Back Perimeter™**: The lower edge of the scalp, from ear to ear across the nape and back hairline.

**Central Line™**: The midline of the scalp running from the front hairline to the back hairline.

**Four Quadrants™**: Four sections divided down the center line and across from ear to ear, over the apex.

**Front Perimeter™**: The border zone framing the forehead and temple area, from in front of the ear to the ear.

**Front Of The Head™:** Area of the scalp from ear to ear over the apex forward to the hairline

**U Section™**: A U-shaped area from the front corners of the hairline, extending back to the crown.

**Top Of The Head™:** The zone of the head from the occipital bone forward to the front perimeter

**Crown**: The upper back portion of the scalp, behind the apex and above the occipital.

**Back**: The area spanning from ear to ear, over the apex, and down to the back hairline.

**Occipital Band™**: The horizontal band beneath the crown and above the nape, extending from behind one ear to the other.

**Nape**: The lowest portion of the scalp, just beneath the occipital bone, extending to the top of the neck.

**Left Side™**: The section between the central line and the left ear, from the front to the back hairline.

**Right Side™**: The section between the central line and the right ear, from the front to the back hairline.

**SSD Evaluation & Execution Framework™**: A methodology designed to guide stylists from consultation through to execution.

**Balanced Distribution™**: A balanced and strategic allocation of weight, shape, color, and tension that complements the client's natural features, hair texture, and scalp landscape.

# 7.
# Consultations & Decision-Making

Through the Lens of the Texture Dynamics Framework™

**The Consultation Journey**

The purpose of a Texture Profile™ is not simply to gather information. The purpose is to make better service providing decisions.

The Texture Profile™ serves as the client's current reality. It captures the characteristics, behaviors, strengths, vulnerabilities, and limitations identified through Hair Properties, Texture Indicators™, Hair Thresholds™, and Scalp Spatial Distribution™. Once documented, the profile becomes the baseline against which all future decisions are measured.

However, a profile alone does not tell us what to do next.

A decision-making protocol must be followed to determine whether a client's goals align with the hair's current capabilities. To accomplish this, the Texture Dynamics Framework™ uses two tools that work together:

- **The Consultation Journey** is the overarching process that guides the appointment from assessment to recommendation.
- **The Service GO / NO-GO Decision Tree** is the evaluation tool used within that process to determine whether the hair can safely tolerate a requested service.

Think of the Consultation Journey as the compass and the Decision Tree as the map. The Journey tells you where you are in the consultation process. The Decision Tree tells you which direction you can safely move. Together, they transform consultation from a subjective conversation into a structured, evidence-based assessment.

The Consultation Journey™ follows six stages: Assess the Hair, Identify the Desired Outcome, Compare Characteristics, Determine Now vs. Journey, Chart the Path, and Deliver Recommendations. The process begins with assessment. Using the Texture Dynamics Framework™, the professional creates a Texture Profile by evaluating the client's Hair Properties, Texture Indicators™, Hair Thresholds™, and Scalp Spatial

Distribution™. These observations are documented on the Texture Profile Wheel™, creating a visual representation of the client's texture profile.

# CONSULTATION JOURNEY

**CHART A PATH TO MORE PERSONALIZED RESULTS.**

A structured approach that ensures every client receives a customized plan rooted in their unique hair needs and goals.

**1 ASSESS THE CLIENT'S HAIR**

- Evaluate the hair's current condition.
- Assess hair properties: density, porosity, elasticity, pattern, scalp condition, and more.
- Document all observations on the TPW.

**2 IDENTIFY CLIENT'S DESIRED STYLE**

- Ask the client what they want to achieve.
- This could be a specific style, texture, length, volume, or overall hair goal.
- Gather references (photos, inspiration) to clarify the vision.

**3 COMPARE CHARACTERISTICS**

- Compare existing hair properties to those presented in the desired style.
- Identify strengths and gaps.
- Note what is needed to bridge the gap.

**4 NOW VS. JOURNEY**

- Determine if the desired style is achievable now.
- Or, does it require a journey (e.g., improving elasticity, increasing length, restoring density)?

**5 CHART THE PATH**

- If it's a journey, create a clear plan.
- Outline the steps, treatments, regimens, and timelines needed to move from point A (now) to point B (goal).

**6 RECOMMENDATIONS**

- Provide personalized product recommendations.
- Suggest regimen adjustments.
- Recommend lifestyle adjustments that support the goal.



The Texture Profile Wheel™ is more than a recordkeeping tool. It transforms observations into a measurable and repeatable system. By documenting characteristics zone by zone, professionals can identify patterns, inconsistencies, strengths, and vulnerabilities across the scalp. Future assessments can then be compared against previous profiles, making progress visible rather than dependent on memory.

The Wheel also serves as a powerful communication tool. Rather than simply telling a client that their hair is fragile, highly porous, or threshold-sensitive, the professional can visually demonstrate where those characteristics exist and explain how they influence service recommendations. This presents recommendations as observable findings, helping build trust and understanding throughout the consultation process.

## TEXTURE PROFILE WHEEL™

Once the Texture Profile™ has been established, the next step is to identify the client's desired outcome. This may be a specific style, greater length retention, increased density, enhanced curl definition, a color transformation, or improved overall hair health. Reference images and detailed discussion help clarify expectations and ensure both the client and professional share the same vision.

The profile and the goal are then compared. This comparison is one of the most important stages of the consultation process. The Texture Profile™ represents the client's current reality. The desired outcome represents the destination. By comparing the two, the professional can identify strengths that support the goal, vulnerabilities that create risk, and gaps that must be addressed before the goal can be achieved safely.

For example, a client may desire waist-length knotless braids but currently exhibits low elasticity and high porosity. Another client may desire a high-lift blonde transformation while demonstrating compromised Chemical Thresholds™ and signs of previous structural damage. In both situations, the comparison reveals not only what the client wants, but what the hair is capable of supporting today.

This comparison leads directly into Stage 4 of the Consultation Journey™: the Service GO / NO-GO Decision.

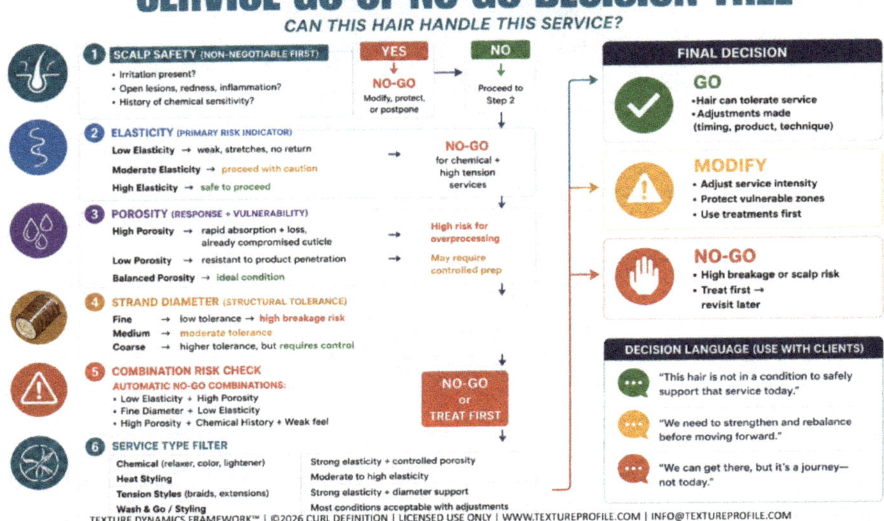


At this stage, the Service GO / NO-GO Decision Tree™ is applied. The Decision Tree serves as the safety gate within the consultation process and is designed to answer a single question:

**Can this hair safely tolerate this service?** The answer determines whether the goal is achievable now, achievable with modifications, or requires a journey.

Ultimately, the most important question in professional consultation is not whether a style can be created. It is whether the hair can safely tolerate the process required to create it. This is where the Texture Dynamics Framework™ shifts the consultation into assessment, styling into strategy, and services into informed decisions that support both beauty and long-term hair integrity.

# 8.
# Aesthetics of Beauty

*Clarifying Aesthetic Goals vs. Natural Traits in Hair Texture Care*

Now that we've explored the complex dynamics of hair textures, it's essential to understand the difference between maximizing a client's natural hair traits and achieving their desired beauty aesthetic.

In its broadest sense, aesthetics refers to the philosophy of beauty and taste, how individuals perceive, experience, and value beauty. In the context of hair, the aesthetics of beauty relate to the visual and tactile attributes that make hair appear appealing: shine, smoothness, curl definition, and more.

However, a client's desired aesthetic may not always align with their natural hair characteristics. For example, a client with fine, low-density coils may desire the appearance of thick, voluminous curls with high definition and shine, traits that aren't naturally present in their texture.

As professionals, our role is to distinguish between the natural traits we aim to enhance and the beauty aesthetics our clients wish to achieve. This requires balancing technical skill, product knowledge, and creativity to bring out the best in their natural texture while getting as close as possible to their desired look, without compromising hair health or long-term growth goals.

## Commonly Desired Hair Aesthetics:

There are certain attributes and qualities that clients commonly aspire to feel and see in their hair. These desired aesthetics include:

- **Shine:** A glossy appearance that reflects light, indicating smooth and well-conditioned hair.
- **Smoothness:** A sleek texture free from frizz and tangles, contributing to a polished look.
- **Softness:** A supple and touchable feel, often associated with healthy hair.
- **Length:** The ability to maintain and grow longer hair without significant breakage.

- **Density:** A full and voluminous appearance, often linked to the thickness and number of hair strands.
- **Consistency in Texture:** Uniformity in hair strand thickness and pattern, leading to a harmonious look.
- **Curl Shape and Definition:** Well-formed curls or waves that are distinct and maintain their pattern.
- **Moisturized:** Hair that retains adequate moisture, preventing dryness and brittleness.
- **Manageability:** Ease of styling and maintaining the desired hairdo without excessive effort.

It's important to recognize that the natural state of one's hair may not inherently possess these desired aesthetics. Factors such as genetics, health, and environmental influences play significant roles in determining hair's natural characteristics. For instance, naturally, curly hair may not exhibit smoothness or shine as prominently as straight hair due to its structure, which can diffuse light differently and be more prone to dryness. Ultimately, our responsibility is to educate, customize our products and methodology, and deliver results that honor the integrity of the hair while enhancing our clients' confidence and satisfaction.

## Achieving Desired Hair Aesthetics:

Combinations of beauty aesthetics requested during salon services often include soft, shiny, long hair with great definition, uniform texture, and extended hold without feeling stiff. While these attributes are often perceived as indicators of healthy hair, they are more often achieved through treatments, salon services, and product applications rather than natural traits. To bridge the gap between natural hair characteristics and desired aesthetics, refer to treatments, salon services, and hair care routines that complement the hair in a way that matches the client's desire:

- **Shine:** Utilize serums or oils that add luster. Regular conditioning treatments can also enhance the hair's reflective quality.

- **Smoothness:** Incorporate smoothing shampoos and conditioners. Professional treatments like keratin can temporarily align hair fibers for a sleeker appearance.

- **Softness:** Deep conditioning masks and leave-in conditioners can infuse moisture, making hair feel softer.
- **Length Retention:** Minimize breakage by reducing heat styling, avoiding harsh chemicals, and regularly trimming split ends.
- **Density:** While genetic factors largely determine density, volumizing products and specific styling techniques can create the illusion of fuller hair.
- **Consistency in Texture:** Chemical treatments or heat styling can temporarily alter texture, but embracing natural patterns with suitable products often yields healthier results.
- **Curl Shape and Definition:** Use curl-enhancing creams or gels and drying techniques like plopping or diffusing to define curls.
- **Moisturized:** Regularly apply hydrating products and avoid over-washing to maintain natural oils.
- **Manageability:** Select hairstyles that complement your natural texture and use detangling products to ease styling.

It's essential to understand that while these methods can enhance the appearance of hair, they may not reflect its underlying health. For example, hair can appear shiny due to silicone-based products without being truly healthy. Therefore, focusing on overall hair health through proper nutrition, gentle handling, and minimizing damaging practices is crucial for authentically achieving and maintaining the desired aesthetics.

This table provides actionable insights to help create or maintain the appearance of desired hair aesthetics, regardless of natural traits. Let me know if you'd like further elaboration on any section.

## Table: Beauty Aesthetic Methodology

| Desired Aesthetic | Natural Trait Needed | Methods to Achieve Aesthetic |
|---|---|---|
| **Length Retention** | Strong hair structure with low breakage and split ends. | Build or maintain elasticity with moisture protein balance, trim ends regularly, and avoid excessive manipulation and heat. Incorporate protective styles when needed. |
| **Density** | High number of hair follicles and naturally thick strands. | Use volumizing products, clip-in extensions, diffuse drying, and scalp-stimulating treatments and growth serums. |
| **Consistency in Texture** | Uniform thickness and texture shape along hair strands. | Use texture-balancing wet sets, bond repair treatments. |
| **Curl Shape** | Well-defined natural curl or wave patterns. | Use curl-defining creams, gels, and mousse; employ styling techniques like diffusing, finger coiling, or perm rods. Accommodate variations of texture shape with blending techniques. |
| **Curl Definition** | Naturally separated and moisturized curls. | Apply curl creams and gels; use Curl Definition method, plopping, or twist-outs to create and maintain texture shape. |
| **Moisturized** | Hair with natural sebum distribution and balanced porosity. | Shampoo weekly, deep condition regularly, use water-based moisturizers, rehydrating mists, lipids, occlusives, sealants oils or butters. |
| **Manageable** | Hair that detangles easily and responds well to styling. | Use detangling sprays, wide-tooth combs, or brushes; incorporate regular deep conditioning and protective styles, keep hair stretched. |

# 9.
# Managing Textured Hair

*A Tailored Approach for Professionals*

Managing hair textures requires a specialized approach that extends beyond standard hair care practices. As a service provider, it is your responsibility not only to understand the unique characteristics of hair textures but also to educate clients on how to care for it properly. This involves implementing techniques and recommending products that preserve the hair's health, enhance its beauty, and respect its natural structure.

**Detangling: The Foundation of Managing Hair Textures**

It is crucial to emphasize detangling as the starting point for healthy hair management. Poor detangling practices are one of the leading causes of breakage, split ends, and compromised hair integrity, especially in tightly textured hair types. Teaching proper detangling techniques and designing products that support gentle, effective detangling are key to preserving the beauty, strength, and longevity of hair textures.

**The Importance of Using the Right Tools**

The first step in effective detangling is selecting appropriate tools. Flexible detangling brushes with wide-spaced, moving bristles, wide-tooth combs, and detangling-specific brushes (like those with staggered bristle heights) are ideal for highly textured hair. These tools minimize tension, reduce snagging, and allow hair to glide through without unnecessary pulling. Tools should always be flexible enough to move with the hair, not against it, helping to prevent mechanical damage to both the strand and the follicle.

**Never Detangle Tightly Textured Hair While Dry**

Detangling tightly textured hair dry is a guaranteed route to unnecessary breakage. Tightly textured hair, especially when dry, lacks the pliability needed to withstand pulling and manipulation. Always teach that tightly textured hair should be detangled on wet or damp hair, preferably saturated with a slip-enhancing product, to allow strands to separate smoothly without excessive friction or tension. If detangling must occur on slightly damp hair (for example, during styling prep), always mist with water and use a leave-in conditioner or a detangling spray to add slip.

## Detangling Products: A Critical Support System

Detangling products are not optional; they are a crucial support system for managing hair textures. Ideal detanglers should provide lubrication, hydration, and softening without heavy buildup. Products like leave-in conditioners, detangling sprays, conditioning mists, and foaming leave-ins are formulated to reduce friction between strands. As product developers, we prioritize ingredients like aloe vera, marshmallow root extract, glycerin, slippery elm, panthenol, and lightweight oils to create effective detangling aids that protect the hair shaft during manipulation.

## The Proper Way to Detangle Hair

Proper technique is just as important as tools and products:

- **Work in Sections:** Always divide the hair into manageable sections before attempting to detangle. Depending on density and length, four to eight sections are often appropriate. Sectioning prevents overwhelm, maintains moisture, and ensures thorough detangling without stressing the hair.
- **Start from the Ends:** Begin detangling at the ends of the hair first. Gently work out knots and tangles a few inches at a time, gradually moving upward toward the roots. Starting from the scalp down can tighten knots, leading to tearing and severe breakage.
- **Keep Hair Moisturized:** Never allow the ends to dry out during detangling. The ends are the oldest and most fragile part of the hair strand, and dry ends are more susceptible to splitting and snapping. If the hair begins to dry while working through sections, mist it lightly with water or reapply your detangling product to maintain elasticity and flexibility.
- **Use Gentle Motions:** Use a gentle, downward motion, gliding the brush or comb through the hair. Avoid yanking or pulling through tangles; instead, work slowly and patiently, encouraging the hair to separate naturally.
- **Use Fingers First if Necessary:** For tighter tangles or matted areas, finger-detangling before using a tool can prevent unnecessary damage. Your fingers can feel knots more sensitively than a comb or brush, allowing for delicate separation of strands.

Another critical aspect of texture care is moisture management. Because of its structure, highly textured hair is inherently drier than straight hair, making it difficult for natural oils to travel down the shaft. Educating clients on the importance of moisture and recommending hydrating products can significantly impact their hair's overall health. Determine how often the client's hair should be shampooed and conditioned on an individual basis. While some clients can go without shampooing between their bi-monthly salon visits, others may require cleansing twice a week. There is no "one size fits all". The frequency of your washes should depend on your hair's unique characteristics, lifestyle, and even the changing seasons. During colder months, environmental dryness can make hair more prone to brittleness, while summer heat may increase sweat and product buildup. Pay attention to how your hair reacts between washes and adjust your routine accordingly. Guide clients on how to maintain clean hair with the proper shampoos and conditioners for their hair needs and the importance of a routine that uses a cycle of gentle cleansers, moisturizing cleansers, and clarifying cleansers. Additionally, select conditioners customized to your clients' hair needs. Tight-textured hair greatly benefits from rich, effective conditioning treatments. Offering deep conditioning services and suggesting leave-in conditioners can help clients lock in moisture, reduce breakage, maintain softness and manageability, and manage hair.

Styling product selection is equally important. Textured hair thrives with heavier, emollient-based formulations that provide lasting hydration and protection. Products that include lipids, occlusives, and oils help seal in moisture, reduce frizz, and add shine. Your expertise in choosing the right products for each client's texture shape, density, porosity, and elasticity sets the foundation for successful outcomes and client satisfaction.

Styling hair textures requires both creativity and technical skill. Mastering styling techniques is vital, so continuing education should always be a part of your portfolio. With a wide array of advanced styling options, professionals can offer customized services that celebrate each client's unique Texture Dynamics™ and style preferences.

Curl definition is a popular goal, achieved through curl-enhancing products and precise techniques. The beauty of working with highly textured hair lies in its versatility and expressive potential. Styling free natural hair includes a variety of techniques to either enhance natural texture or create new patterns. Creating texture through twist-outs and braid-outs, creating curl patterns using finger coils, comb coils, rod sets, or roller sets, and defining the natural curl pattern through wash-and-gos, curl training, or curl definition methods gives clients countless options to express themselves.

Protective styles such as braids and twists not only look beautiful but also reduce manipulation and help maintain hair health. For clients who prefer a straighter look, thermal straightening can be offered, but it is critical to use modern tools and stress the importance of heat protection. Extensions and wigs offer even more versatility, allowing clients to explore different looks, add volume, or protect their natural hair. Guiding clients in choosing and maintaining wigs as a protective style can further strengthen your role as a knowledgeable and trusted professional.

Preserving the delicate nature of highly textured hair is another essential component of care. Gentle detangling, minimizing heat, and using silk or satin accessories are just a few methods that help maintain the integrity of hair textures. Clients should be educated on protection from environmental stressors, such as sun exposure and harsh weather, using UV-protective products and protective styles. Preservation involves maintaining the natural texture shape and avoiding excessive manipulation between salon visits. Equipping clients with the right tools and at-home care routines fosters independence and strengthens your professional relationship. Building strength through protein treatments and fortifying products helps reinforce the hair shaft, reducing breakage and promoting resilience.

An expert eye is also needed to identify and address early signs of damage. Common issues such as single-strand knots, loss of curl integrity, split strands, and loss of elasticity should be handled with care. Educate clients on preventive measures like regular trims, proper detangling, and restorative treatments. Offer professional solutions that target specific damage while promoting long-term health and strength.

Ultimately, the key to delivering exceptional service lies in shifting from a one-size-fits-all method to a more tailored, comprehensive approach that addresses each client's individual needs. Understanding the nuances of hair textures, whether curly, coily, or kinky, enables you to elevate your practice, build trust, and empower clients to embrace their natural beauty with confidence. Your dedication to specialized care, continuous education, and personalized service will position you as a leader in the texture care industry.

## Foundational Product Guide - Based On Texture Dynamics

Selecting the right products for hair care and styling starts with understanding the hair's Texture State, which includes three key components: texture shape (straight, wavy, curly, coily/kinky, or incongruent), strand diameter (fine, medium, or thick), and hair properties (porosity, density, elasticity, and shrinkage). These factors work together to determine how hair absorbs and retains moisture, maintains volume, responds to styling, and holds curl patterns. Without considering these unique characteristics, it becomes difficult to maintain healthy, manageable hair. Below is a guide to help tailor your hair care and styling routine according to these defining features.

Straight hair often requires lightweight hydration and volume support, especially for finer strands. Fine straight hair with low porosity benefits from clarifying shampoos to remove buildup and mist-based conditioners with humectants like aloe vera. If porosity is high, protein-infused conditioners and light serums help strengthen and seal the cuticle. Low-density straight hair thrives on volumizing foams, while high-density strands may need lightweight serums for frizz control. Elasticity plays a key role; strengthening protein treatments are ideal when it's low. Recommended products include sulfate-free volumizing shampoos, silk-protein conditioners, and mousses or serums for body and shine. Medium strands require hydration with ingredients like coconut water or panthenol, and deep-conditioning masks for high porosity. Depending on density and elasticity, smoothing creams and volumizing mousse are ideal stylers. Thick straight strands benefit from weekly clarifying to reduce buildup, and deep conditioners rich in protein, paired with smoothing serums or protectant sprays.

Wavy hair needs moisture without weight to preserve its natural flow. Fine, wavy hair with low porosity thrives on mist conditioners, while high porosity hair needs protein-rich masks to restore structure. Lightweight foams suit low-density hair, and medium-hold creams define high-density waves. When elasticity is low, flexible hold sprays support style longevity. Medium strands require water-based leave-ins for hydration and curl refreshers to maintain definition without build-up. For thick, wavy hair, deep hydration and sealing butters, such as shea or mango, help prevent moisture loss. Low-density waves need flexible creams, while high-density strands benefit from strong-hold gels. Suggested cleansers range from gentle shampoos to rich moisture conditioners, with stylers like curl creams, mousses, and humidity-resistant sprays.

Curly hair demands consistent moisture, curl enhancement, and frizz control. Fine curly hair with low porosity responds well to hydrating mists and lightweight leave-ins, while high porosity curls benefit from cream-based leave-ins and protein treatments. Volumizing curl foams suit low-density curls, while soft-hold gels define thicker sets without stiffness. Medium curly strands do best with creamy leave-ins and deep conditioning treatments containing ceramides. Stylers like defining creams or flexible-hold gels help maintain the curl pattern. Thick strands often need water-based creams for hydration and butters to seal moisture. For density, lighter stylers prevent weight on low-density curls, while firm gels or custards control high-density curls. Recommended products include co-washes, sulfate-free cleansers, protein-rich deep conditioners, and defining stylers customized to thickness and texture.

Coily and kinky hair has the greatest need for moisture retention, structural support, and protective care. Fine, coily hair with low porosity benefits from spritz-based hydrators and light leave-ins, while high porosity strands require rich creams and oils for layered moisture. Curl creams enhance fullness for low-density hair, while custards define coils in higher densities without causing stiffness. Medium and thick coily strands need pre-poo treatments for better moisture absorption and benefit from layering butters and creams to lock hydration. Styling depends on density, lightweight creams for low-density coils, and heavier custards or strong-hold gels for high-density textures. Suggested products include moisturizing cleansers or co-washes, intensive hydrating masks, and styling products that offer control without compromising flexibility.

# GLOSSARY / INDEX

## HOW TO READ THIS GLOSSARY

* Terms original to the Texture Profile Framework™, coined by the author.

** Industry terms redefined within this framework. A conventional reference is included beneath the entry.

*** Industry terms applied in a specialized or expanded way within this framework.

No marker, standard industry term used in its conventional sense.

*Terms marked *, **, or *** are the intellectual property of the author. Use of these terms in educational curricula, commercial materials, publications, or professional training programs requires written licensure from the author. Licensing inquiries: info@textureprofile.com*

**A**

**Acidic:** A pH below 7. *p. 105*

**Alkaline:** A pH above 7 . *p. 105*

**Altered Hair™**: The state in which one or more thresholds are exceeded, resetting the hair's shape while preserving its internal structure. *p. 63**

**Altered State™:** The state in which one or more thresholds are exceeded, resetting the hair's shape while preserving its internal structure. p. 118*

**Altered Texture™**: A Texture Recovery™ outcome in which the hair does not return to its original pattern but remains structurally sound in an Altered State™, retaining flexibility and resilience in a new configuration. *p. 104**

**Anagen**: The active phase of the Growth Cycle. *p. 51*

**Anchors™**: The Front Hair Line, Back Hair Line, and Central Line that act as reference markers. *p. 130**

**Angle of Emergence™**: The general angle at which hair exits the scalp. *p. 70****

*Conventional use:* *Appears in hair transplant surgery and biology literature but not in standard cosmetology. Applied here as a cosmetology assessment tool within the Texture Profile Framework™.*

**Apex**: The highest point of the head, located at the top-center of the head. *p. 127*

**Atmospheric Heat™**: A distribution of heat into the atmosphere surrounding the hair. *p. 99**

**B**

**Back**: The area spanning from ear to ear, over the apex, and down to the back hairline. *p. 135*

**Back Hair Line™**: The lower boundary of the scalp at the nape, extending from behind one ear to the other. *p. 129**

**Back Perimeter™**: The lower edge of the scalp, from ear to ear across the nape and back hairline. *p. 134**

**Balanced Distribution™**: A balanced and strategic allocation of weight, shape, color, and tension that complements the client's natural features, hair texture, and scalp landscape. *p. 148****

*Conventional use:* *Balance is a standard design principle. This framework applies it as a unified, multi-discipline strategic concept.*

**Balanced Integrity™:** Hair that demonstrates a stable and predictable response to chemical processing while maintaining manageable elasticity, structural resilience, and recoverability. p. 104*

**Branched Splits™**: A slivered or tapered shortened strand end resembling a tree branch. *p. 111**

## C

**Catagen**: The resting phase of the Growth Cycle. *p. 51*

**Central Line™**: The midline of the scalp running from the front hairline to the back hairline. *p. 129**

**Chemical burns**: Injuries caused by excessive chemical exposure to the skin or scalp. *p. 108*

**Chemical Threshold™**: The hair's ability to tolerate chemical-induced structural alteration before the integrity of the fiber becomes compromised. p. 103*

**Coily Hair**: Hair with tight corkscrew, helix, or "O" shaped curls. *p. 73*

**Compromised Integrity™:** Hair that has reduced structural stability and increased vulnerability due to repeated stress, excessive processing, cumulative threshold exceedance, or chronic environmental and mechanical damage. p. 105*

**Compromised Texture™**: The Texture Recovery outcome in which the hair loses its ability to maintain a consistent or recognizable pattern due to structural disruption from exceeded thresholds. *p. 118**

**Corners of the Hair Line™**: The left and right points of the front hairline, between the central line and the temple zone, where the hairline changes direction, and the outermost points where the back hairline meets the nape boundary, functioning as reference markers that establish balance, guide sectioning, and align placement across styling, cutting, and coloring services. *p. 128****

> ***Conventional use:** Standard cosmetology identifies four corners as structural points where the head changes from flat to round, used in haircutting geometry. The TPF™ defines front and back corners as distinct, separately located navigational markers.*

**Cortex**: The middle layer of the hair, containing melanin pigment and fibrous protein. *p. 25*

**Crown**: The upper back portion of the scalp, behind the apex and above the occipital. *p. 132*

**Curl Pattern™**: When the Texture Shape is consistent and uniform along the length of the hair. *p. 74***

> ***Conventional use:*** *Industry use: The general wave or curl configuration of the hair, often described by curl type systems.*

**Curly Hair**: Hair with spirals or loops, ranging from loose, bouncy curls to tighter ringlets, with defined "S" or "O" shapes. *p. 731*

**Cuticle**: The outermost layer of the hair. *p. 25*

## D

**Damaged State™**: The condition of hair in which structural integrity has been disrupted due to threshold exceedance, resulting in incongruent texture, weakness, brittleness, or loss of pattern. *p. 118**

**Degree of Shrinkage™**: The difference between the hair's True Length and its Perceived Length when the hair contracts to its natural texture shape. *p. 47**

**Density**: The number of hair strands per square inch of the scalp. *p. 37*

**Direct Heat™**: The immediate transfer of heat from the heat source to the hair's surface. *p. 99****

> ***Conventional use:*** *Industry use: Used broadly to mean any tool-applied heat. Applied here as a precise category within the TPF™ five-part heat delivery typology.*

**Disulfide Bonds**: Very strong bonds that can only be changed with chemicals like relaxers, perms, or bleach, or extreme heat. *p. 26*

## E

**Elasticity**: The hair's ability to stretch and return to its original shape without breaking. *p. 31*

**Excessive Shedding™**: Hair shedding that goes beyond the normal daily loss of 50–100 strands. *p. 111**

## F

**Four Quadrants™**: Four sections divided down the center line and across from ear to ear, over the apex. *p. 130***

> ***Conventional use:*** *Industry use: Sectioning is a standard technique but is not mapped as a named spatial zone. This framework defines Four Quadrants as a foundational zone structure within Scalp Spatial Distribution™.*

**Fractured Cuticles™**: A small, bare section on the strand where the cuticle layer has been stripped away. *p. 111**

**Friction Threshold™**: The hair's ability to withstand repeated physical interaction with materials. *p. 116**

**Front**: The area spanning from ear to ear, over the apex, and forward to the front hairline. *p. 131*

**Front Corners:** The area of the front hairline, which mark the transition from the center of the hairline to the temples, which mark the transition from the center of the hairline to the temples. *p. 127*

**Front Hair Line™**: The edge of the scalp above the forehead, spanning from temple to temple. *p. 129****

> ***Conventional use:*** *Industry use: Referenced as a hairline boundary. Applied here as a named navigational anchor within Scalp Spatial Distribution™.*

**Front Of The Head™:** Area of the scalp from ear to ear over the apex forward to the hairline. P. 130

**Front Perimeter™**: The border zone framing the forehead and temple area, from in front of the ear to the ear. *p. 130**

## G

**Growth Rate™**: The rate at which an individual's hair grows. *p. 51*

## H

**Hair**: A thread-like filament of dead, keratinized protein cells that grow from follicles in the scalp. *p. 25*

**Hair Bulb**: The structure of the hair that forms the lower part of the hair root. *p. 25*

**Hair Follicle**: The structure of the hair that holds the hair root. *p. 25*

**Hair Properties™**: Specific hair traits that determine hair's appearance, behavior, and overall health, including Elasticity, Density, Porosity, and Length. *p. 31****

> ***Conventional use:*** *Industry use: Hair properties are referenced generally. This framework defines a specific, bounded set of four properties as a pillar of the Texture Dynamics Framework™.*

**Hair Root**: The structure of the hair enclosed within the follicle beneath the skin surface. *p. 25*

**Hair Shaft**: The structure of the hair that extends beyond the skin surface. *p. 26*

**Hair Texture™**: The overall appearance and tactile experience of the hair, encompassing the shape, movement, and feel of the hair. *p. 26***

> ***Conventional use:*** *Industry use: In standard cosmetology, hair texture refers to the diameter of the individual strand; fine, medium, or coarse.*

**Hair Thresholds™**: The tolerance limit that hair has for various external stressors and internal deficiencies. *p. 83**

**Heat Damage™**: The result of when hair's heat threshold is exceeded. *p. 98****

**Heat Delivery™**: How heat is administered to hair during a service. *p. 98**

> ***Conventional use:*** *Industry use: Describes visible damage from heat. Applied here as a threshold-linked outcome within the TPF™ heat framework.*

**Heat Response™**: How the hair responds to exposure to heat. *p. 95**

**Heat Threshold™**: The point at which hair can no longer endure thermal exposure without experiencing structural changes. *p. 95**

**Heat Training™**: The controlled use of moderate heat over time to loosen the natural texture. *p. 97****

> ***Conventional use:*** *Industry use: Used broadly without a framework-based definition or threshold relationship.*

**High Resistance™:** Hair that demonstrates a stronger ability to maintain structural stability during chemical services and typically resists rapid chemical penetration. P. 104*

**Hydration**: The act of increasing the hair's water content. *p. 89*

**Hydrogen Bonds**: Weak bonds that can easily be broken with water or heat. *p. 25*

**Hygral Fatigue**: Weakening of the hair as it undergoes repeated swelling and contracting due to excessive moisture. *p. 91*

**I**

**Incongruent Texture™**: Hair with a Texture Shape that lacks consistency or repetition along the strand, displaying no discernible pattern at all. p. 73 *

**Incongruent Texture Shape™**: Hair that bends and curves in primarily frizzy or wiry movement without a distinct curl or wave formation, and often appears unruly.

p. 73 *

**Ionic Influenced Heat™**: A heat distribution that involves applying heat while releasing negative ions to break water molecules into smaller particles. *p. 100**

**K**

**Kinky Hair™**: Hair with tight, sharp bends and zigzag forms. *p. 72****

> ***Conventional use:*** *Industry use: Used inconsistently and sometimes avoided. This framework establishes it as a precise structural hair form classification.*

**L**

**Left Side™**: The section between the central line and the left ear, from the front to the back hairline. *p. 135**

**Length**: The measurement of hair from root to end. *p. 47*

**Length Retention™**: The ability to preserve hair length. *p. 52****

***Conventional use:*** *Industry use: Used informally in the natural hair community without a clinical definition. Applied here as a measurable, framework-linked outcome.*

M

**Manipulation Threshold™**: The maximum mechanical stress and product application that the hair and follicles can endure. *p. 110**

**Mastoid Process**: A bony protrusion located just behind the earlobe. *p. 127*

**Mechanical Stress™**: All types of physical forces applied to the hair and scalp. *p. 108***

***Conventional use:*** *Industry use: Referenced broadly across disciplines. Applied here as a bounded, threshold-linked concept.*

**Medulla**: The innermost layer of the hair, composed of round cells containing mainly airspace. *p. 25*

**Moisture Cycle™**: The natural process in which hair absorbs, retains, and loses moisture over time. *p. 93**

**Moisture Level™**: The amount of water content within the hair strands. *p.,32, 90****

***Conventional use:*** *Industry use: Referenced generally. Applied here as a measurable state within the TPF™ moisture framework.*

**Moisture Retention Regimen™**: A routine of layering hydrators and moisturizers to maintain a healthy moisture level. *p. 93**

**Moisture Threshold™**: The maximum level of hydration or moisture loss that hair can absorb without compromising its structural integrity. *p. 87**

**Moisturization™**: The process of sealing and protecting hydration by forming a barrier around the hair strand. *p. 89***

> ***Conventional use:*** *Industry use: Often used interchangeably with hydration. This framework distinguishes moisturization and hydration as two distinct, sequential processes.*

## N

**Nape**: The lowest portion of the scalp, just beneath the occipital bone, extending to the top of the neck. *p. 134*

**Natural Fall™**: The way hair naturally positions itself in response to gravity based on its inherent Texture Shape and Angle of Emergence. *p. 70****

> ***Conventional use:*** *Industry use: Referenced in haircutting as 'natural falling position.' Applied here as a defined characteristic linked to Texture Shape™ and Angle of Emergence™.*

**Natural Hair™**: Hair that retains its original structure and characteristics. *p. 65***

> ***Conventional use:*** *Industry use: Used culturally and informally. This framework defines it structurally in direct contrast to Altered Hair™.*

**Natural State™**: The condition of hair that retains its original structure, Texture Shape™, and Texture Pattern™ without permanent deviation. *p. 118**

**Needle-Eye Split**: A small, isolated slit anywhere along the hair shaft. *p. 111*

**Neutral:** A pH of 7. *p. 105*

## O

**Occipital Band™**: The horizontal band beneath the crown and above the nape, extending from behind one ear to the other. *p. 127**

**Occipital Region**: The rounded lower back portion of the skull, centered around the occipital bone. *p. 127*

**Overexposure:** When the hair or scalp is subjected to a chemical process beyond its tolerance level. .*p. 107*

**P**

**Parietal Ridge**: The curved lateral section of the head that runs from the top of the ear upward toward the crown. *p. 127*

**Perceived Length™**: How long the hair appears when it rests in its texture shape. *p. 47**

**Perpetual Motion™**: The continuous, responsive movement of hair as it expands, contracts, and reshapes itself. *p. 71**

**pH, or "Potential Hydrogen":** Measures how acidic or alkaline a substance is on a scale from 0 to 14. *p. 105*

**Porosity**: The hair's ability to absorb, retain, and release moisture. *p. 40*

**Protein Level™**: The amount and quality of keratin and other structural proteins present in the cortex. *p. 32**

**Protein Overload™**: When hair exceeds its protein threshold. *p. 86****

> ***Conventional use:*** *Industry use: Described informally. Applied here as a threshold-linked outcome within the TPF™ protein framework.*

**Protein State™**: The condition of the hair as a result of its protein levels. *p. 85**

**Protein Threshold™**: The maximum amount of protein your hair can absorb before it starts to experience adverse effects. *p. 84**

## R

**Radiant Heat™**: A distribution of infrared heat that increases penetration by warming the hair from within. *p. 9100**

**Recovered Texture™**: A Texture Recovery™ outcome in which the hair returns fully to its Natural State™, maintaining its Texture Shape™ and Texture Pattern™ after a service, indicating thresholds were respected and internal structure remains intact. *p. 118**

**Right Side™**: The section between the central line and the right ear, from the front to the back hairline. *p. 135**

## S

**Salt Bonds**: Hair bonds formed between positive and negative charges that are easily broken by changes in pH. *p. 26*

**Scalp Spatial Distribution (SSD)™**: A trait-based method of mapping the scalp that enables stylists to deliver customized, precision-based hair care. *p. 128**

**Sealants™**: Hydrophobic (water-repelling) substances that create a protective barrier over the hair shaft. *p. 89***

> ***Conventional use:*** *Industry use: Used interchangeably with moisturizers and conditioners. This framework defines sealants as a distinct functional category.*

**Shrinkage™**: The natural phenomenon in which textured hair contracts and appears shorter than its true length when fully stretched or straightened. *p. 47**

**Sideburns**: The vertical area that extends from the temple region down to the jawline, located in front of the ear. *p. 127*

**Single-Strand Knots**: Tiny knots formed by tangles in individual strands. *p. 112*

**Split End**: The hair strand divides at the tip in a "Y" shape. *p. 110*

**SSD Evaluation & Execution Framework™**: A methodology designed to guide stylists from consultation through to execution. *p. 135**

**SSD Service Plan™**: A diagramed, customized, region-specific strategy for delivering hair services, guided by Scalp Spatial Distribution mapping. *p. 135**

**Steam Heat™**: A heat distribution that introduces warmth alongside water vapor, allowing the hair to expand rather than contract. *p. 97**

**Straight Hair**: Hair that lacks natural bends or curves and falls uniformly from the scalp. *p. 73*

**Straight Natural™**: Hair that has had its texture shape permanently altered without exposure to chemicals, normally through thermal straightening. *p. 68**

**Strand Diameter™**: The width of an individual strand of hair. *p. 54**

## T

**Telogen**: The resting phase of the Growth Cycle. *p. 51*

**Temple**: The area between the end of the eyebrows and the top of the ears, forward of the parietal ridge. *p. 130*

**Tension Threshold™**: The point at which a hair fiber can be stretched or elongated without compromising its structural integrity. *p. 110**

**Texture Dynamics Framework™**: A comprehensive approach to identifying, understanding, and caring for an individual's unique hair traits by use of a personalized tri-layered assessment of Hair Properties, Texture Dynamics, and Hair Thresholds. *p. 23**

**Texture Feel™**: The tactile feel and appearance of hair. *p. 75**

**Texture Indicators™**: The various hair characteristics that interact and work together to influence the Hair Texture. *p. 65**

**Texture Movement™**: Hair's constant state of motion as it emerges from the scalp to bend, turn, and curve to create shape and patterns. *p. 70**

**Texture Movement Spectrum™**: The full range of variable movement that hair expresses, from tightly coiled to completely straight and incongruent, encompassing Texture Shape™ and Texture Pattern™, with no single texture as the default. *p. 720**

**Texture Pattern™**: Represents how the Texture Shape repeats along the length of the hair strand. *p. 74**

**Texture Profile Wheel™**: A hair analysis tool that evaluates the complexity of each individual's hair texture. *p. 24**

**Texture Recovery™**: The hair's response to a service, assessed by whether the hair returns to, adapts from, or is unable to reestablish its natural Texture Shape™ and Texture Pattern™. *p. 117**

**Texture Shape™**: The form and curvature of a hair strand and where it lies within the Texture Movement Spectrum™, ranging from tightly coiled to straight or frizzy. *p. 72**

**Texture State™**: The classification of hair's current condition in relation to its original structure, Natural State™, Altered State™, or Damaged State™, reflecting where the hair exists in its overall journey at any given point in time. *p. 65**

**Three Pillars of Hair™**: Hair Properties, Texture Indicators, and Hair Thresholds. *p. 23**

**Top™**: The area from the apex forward to the front perimeter, between the parietal ridges. *p. 132****

> ***Conventional use:*** *Standard zone designation. Boundaries here are defined by TPF™ proprietary reference points, including Front Perimeter™.*

**Top Of The Head™**: The zone of the head from the occipital bone forward to the front perimeter. *p. 132**

**Transitioning Hair™**: Hair in a mixed state, where natural texture is growing at the roots, but altered hair remains on the ends. *p. 66**

**True Length™**: The actual full length of hair strands when completely extended or straightened. *p. 47**

U

**U Section™**: A U-shaped area from the front corners of the hairline, extending back to the crown. *p. 131**

**Unaltered Response™**: The state of hair in which there is no permanent change to the hair's structure from thermal exposure, and it easily reverts to its original natural texture shape without lasting effects. *p. 975**

**Wavy Hair**: Hair that is characterized by loose, flowing "S" shapes, moving in gentle undulations. *p. 73*

# APPENDIX

## TEXTURE PROFILE WHEEL™ ASSESSMENT

*Select the dots that identifies the hair characteristic.*

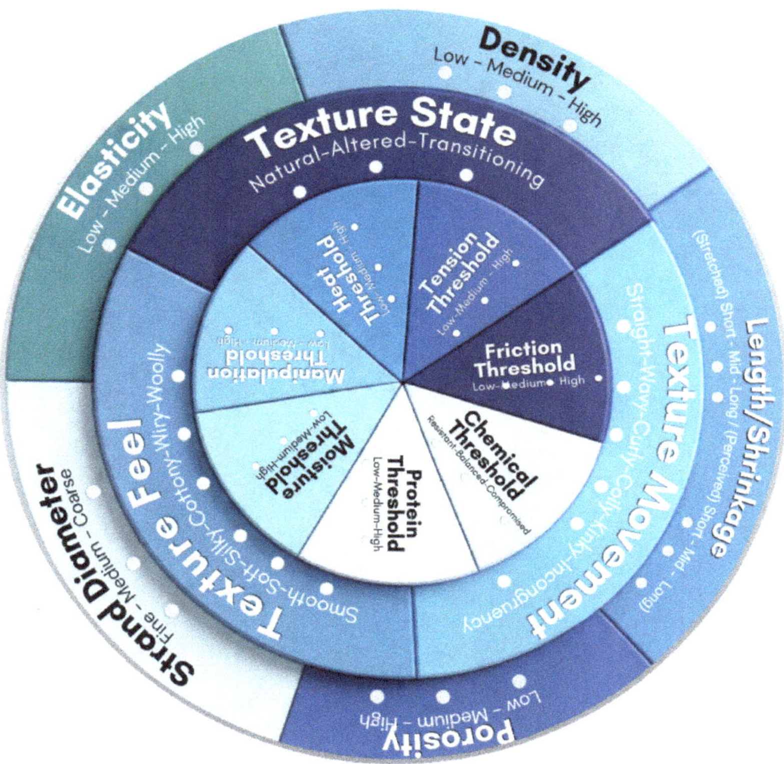


## TEXTURE MOVEMENT SPECTRUM™

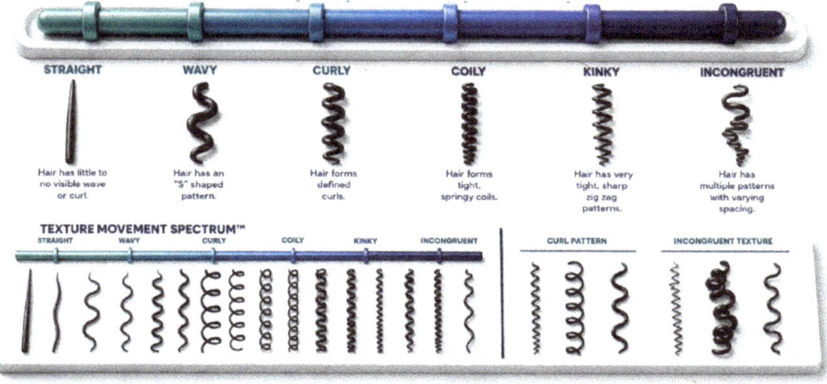

# PROTEIN THRESHOLD DIAGNOSTIC

## Protein Threshold Diagnostic Table

This table is designed to assess the Protein Threshold of hair, which determines how much protein reinforcement a strand can tolerate before it becomes brittle or unbalanced. Use this tool to evaluate the hair's need for protein, its reaction to treatments, and the risk of over-proteinization. Each category is rated from 1 (Low Threshold) to 3 (High Threshold) based on observable behavior during and after care.

**How to Use the Table:**

1. Perform a pre-assessment of the Hair Properties and Texture Indicators on freshly cleansed, product-free hair.
2. Perform a post-assessment on treated hair, prior to the styling session.
3. Evaluate the hair across each category: Protein Absorption, Hair Properties, Texture Indicators with special attention to elasticity response.
4. During styling, note any unusual hair Behavior.
5. Use results to guide product selection and treatment frequency, balancing with moisture as needed.

| Identifier | 1 – Low Threshold | 2 – Medium Threshold | 3 – High Threshold |
| --- | --- | --- | --- |
| **Protein Absorption** | Hair resists protein products or feels stiff/rough immediately after application and moisture treatment doesn't resolve. | Hair absorbs light-to-moderate protein well and shows mild improvement in strength and structure. | Hair readily accepts protein, shows immediate improvement in strength and structure, and feels more stable after use. |
| **Elasticity Response** | Hair snaps when stretched, with little elasticity. | Hair stretches and returns to shape with minimal breakage, indicating balanced elasticity. | Hair has increased stretch and returns to natural texture shape with no signs of brittleness. |
| **Treatment Behavior** | Hair becomes brittle, stiff, or breaks more easily after protein treatments; benefits more from hydration-focused care. | Hair tolerates routine protein use and maintains strength and flexibility when balanced with moisture. | Hair thrives with regular protein treatments and depends on reinforcement to stay resilient and healthy. |

Note: *Always consider porosity, strand diameter, and previous chemical exposure when interpreting protein needs. Reassess threshold levels regularly, especially after periods of breakage, chemical services, or seasonal changes.*

# MOISTURE THRESHOLD DIAGNOSTIC

## Moisture Threshold Diagnostic Table

This table helps determine hair's Moisture Threshold by scoring five key identifiers. Each indicator is rated from 1 (Low Moisture Threshold) to 3 (High Moisture Threshold). Total the points to assess the appropriate care strategy.

| Identifier | 1 – Low Threshold | 2 – Medium Threshold | 3 – High Threshold |
|---|---|---|---|
| **Absorption Speed** | Absorbs instantly, dries quickly. | Absorbs moderately. | Repels water; takes time to absorb. |
| **Moisture Retention** | Feels dry by Day 1–2, before needing moisturization. | Feels moisturized 3–4 days before needing moisturization. | Stays moisturized 5+ days or resists moisturization. |
| **Hydration Response** | Immediately hydrates, softens or swells. | Hydrates within 2–3 min. | Requires 3+ min to hydrate; heat may be needed. |
| **Signs Hydration Level Surpassed** | Mussy, limp, stretchy to the point of breakage. | Mussy, limp, stretchy to the point of breakage. | Mussy, limp, stretchy to the point of breakage. |
| **Signs of Excessive Moisture Loss** | Frizz, tangles easily, dull, rough, does not hold styles. | Frizz, tangles easily, dull, rough, does not hold styles. | Resistant, stiff, rough, lacking curl definition. |

# HEAT THRESHOLD LEVELS

## Heat Threshold Diagnostic Table

This table is designed to assess the Heat Threshold level of hair, its ability to tolerate thermal styling without experiencing structural damage or irreversible changes. Use this tool to evaluate how hair responds to heat based on its porosity, elasticity, strand diameter, and hair health. Each identifier is rated from 1 (Low Threshold) to 3 (High Threshold) based on real-time behavior and post-heat effects.

### How to Use the Table:

1. Pre-assess the Hair Properties and Texture Indicators before thermal styling.
2. Perform a post-assessment on freshly washed hair, immediately following a heat styling session.
3. Evaluate the hair across each category: Hair Properties, texture Indicators, and Texture Recovery.
4. Determine if treatments and/or a trim is necessary to preserve hair health or set a journey to repair.

| Identifier | 1 – Low Threshold | 2 – Medium Threshold | 3 – High Threshold |
|---|---|---|---|
| **Texture Recovery** | Texture Shape and/or Texture Pattern does not return or is significantly looser after one or two heat applications; texture appears altered or limp. | Texture Shape and/or Texture Pattern gradually returns after wash with minimal textural change; slight elongation may be visible, or hair is permanently straightened without the integrity of the hair being compromised. | Curl pattern snaps back fully with no visible change; strong texture memory even after repeated heat use. |
| **Hair Behavior** | Hair feels weak or limp after thermal service or blow-drying; breakage may increase noticeably. | Hair feels slightly dry but manageable; retains softness and strength with proper care. | Hair remains soft, pliable, and resilient post-heat with no signs of stress or dryness. |

Note: *Heat thresholds may vary across zones of the scalp. Always reassess threshold levels before increasing frequency or temperature of thermal styling, and incorporate proper thermal protection and recovery strategies to preserve curl integrity and fiber strength. Protein and Bond Repair may be used to support heat recovery.*

# MECHANICAL THRESHOLD DIAGNOSTIC

## Mechanical Threshold Diagnostic Table

This table assesses the Mechanical Thresholds of hair in three key areas: Tension, Manipulation, and Friction. Each category is rated from 1 (Low Threshold) to 3 (High Threshold) based on observable hair responses to mechanical stress. Use this tool to help customize care routines, style choices, and protective strategies based on the hair's mechanical tolerance.

**How to Use the Rubric:**

1. Observe the hair in real-time during detangling, styling, or routine care.
2. Review each category, Tension, Manipulation, and Friction, and choose the score (1, 2, or 3) that best describes the hair's response.
3. Record the finding for each area and identify the lowest-scoring threshold. This is the area most in need of protection or strategy adjustment.
4. Reassess periodically, especially after chemical services, heat exposure, or seasonal changes.
5. Use findings to inform protective styling methods, tool selection, and product application strategies tailored to the client's mechanical profile.

| Identifiers | 1 – Low Threshold | 2 – Medium Threshold | 3 – High Threshold |
|---|---|---|---|
| **Tension Response** | Hair or scalp is sensitive to tension; styles like braids or ponytails cause soreness, thinning, breakage or curl pattern loss in the areas that hair is repeatedly pulled or smoothed. | Hair can tolerate moderate tension without visible stress; shows little to no signs of stress or discomfort. | Hair shows little to no signs of stress with frequent high-tension styles; scalp and strands remain stable. |
| **Manipulation Response** | Hair becomes frizzy, tangled, or breaks easily with moderate combing, brushing, or styling. Hair develops excessive knots. | Hair can handle regular gentle styling and detangling with minimal damage. | Hair remains intact and healthy with frequent manipulation; resists tangling and breakage. |
| **Friction Response** | Hair is highly reactive to surface friction, frizzes easily, or easily shows damage from wigs, synthetics hair, hats, scarves, or cotton pillowcases. | Hair tolerates some friction but benefits from protective fabrics and handling. | Hair resists friction-related damage and maintains structure even with exposure to rougher surfaces. |

Note: *Hair may present different thresholds across various zones of the scalp. Use this rubric in conjunction with visual, tactile, and behavioral assessments to support more precise and individualized care planning.*

# CHEMICAL THRESHOLD DIAGNOSTIC TABLE

This table is designed to help professionals evaluate the relationship between the hair's structural integrity, resistance to chemical alteration, and overall ability to safely tolerate chemical services. Rather than viewing chemical processing as simply "healthy" or "damaged," this table recognizes that hair exists across a spectrum of resistance, stability, and vulnerability. By assessing structural characteristics, visual indicators, processing behavior, and associated risks, professionals can better predict how the hair may respond to services such as coloring, lightening, relaxing, texturizing, permanent waving, or smoothing treatments.

**How to Use the Table:**

1. Create a full Texture Profile by assessing the 3 Pillars of Hair: Hair Properties, Texture Indicators and the other Hair Thresholds
2. Compare your observations to the "Structural Characteristics" and "Common Visual & Physical Indicators" columns to determine threshold range alignment.
3. Review the "Processing Behavior" column to anticipate how the hair is likely to respond during chemical alteration.

| Chemical Threshold™ Range | Structural Characteristics | Common Visual & Physical Indicators | Processing Behavior |
|---|---|---|---|
| **High Resistance™** | Strong structural stability with slower chemical penetration and greater resistance to pH disruption | Compact cuticle appearance, resistant grays, coarse strands, lower porosity tendencies, strong elasticity retention | • **Penetration Speed:** Slow chemical penetration<br>• **Swelling Response:** Controlled to moderate swelling response during processing<br>• **Lift Behavior:** Slower lift or softening behavior that may require strategic saturation, formulation adjustments, or extended timing<br>• **Elasticity Retention:** Maintains elasticity and structural stability longer during controlled processing |
| **Balanced Integrity™** | Stable structural integrity with predictable chemical response and recoverability | Moderate porosity, balanced elasticity, smooth to slightly raised cuticle, consistent texture response | • **Penetration Speed:** Moderate and predictable penetration speed<br>• **Swelling Response:** Balanced swelling response with manageable expansion of the fiber<br>• **Lift Behavior:** Consistent and predictable lift, deposit, or restructuring behavior<br>• **Elasticity Retention:** Maintains stable elasticity and recoverability when processed appropriately |
| **Compromised Integrity™** | Reduced structural stability with weakened resistance to chemical alteration | High porosity, mushy or brittle feel, excessive dryness, cuticle erosion, thinning ends, inconsistent elasticity | • **Penetration Speed:** Rapid and often uneven chemical penetration<br>• **Swelling Response:** Excessive or unstable swelling response that may weaken the fiber further during processing<br>• **Lift Behavior:** Fast, uneven, or unpredictable lift with increased overprocessing risk<br>• **Elasticity Retention:** Higher likelihood of elasticity collapse, fragility, or breakage during processing |

# CLEANSING COMMON INGREDIENTS

| CLEANSING CHEMISTRY | | | | |
|---|---|---|---|---|
| **Product Type** | **Purpose** | **Common Active Ingredients** | **pH** | **Effect on Hair** |
| Clarifying Shampoo | Removes buildup/oils | Sodium C14-16 Olefin Sulfonate, ACV | 5–7 | Slightly swells cuticle |
| Chelating Shampoo | Removes minerals/metals | Disodium EDTA, Tetrasodium EDTA, Citric Acid Phytic Acid | 5–7 | Improves product penetration |
| Moisturizing Shampoo | Gentle cleansing | Cocamidopropyl Betaine, Aloe Vera | 4.5–6 | Supports cuticle balance |
| Surfactants | Lift dirt/oils | Sodium Lauryl Sulfate, Sodium Laureth Sulfate, Cocamidopropyl Betaine | Variable | Cleansing action |

# CONDITIONING & MOISTURE CHEMISTRY

| CONDITIONING & MOISTURE CHEMISTRY | | | | |
|---|---|---|---|---|
| **Product Type** | **Purpose** | **Common Active Ingredients** | **pH** | **Effect on Hair** |
| Conditioners | Smooth cuticle | Behentrimonium Methosulfate, Cetyl Alcohol, Stearyl Alcohol | 3.5–5.5 | Reduces friction |
| Leave-In Conditioners | Ongoing hydration | Panthenol, Aloe Vera, Glycerin | 4–6 | Improves flexibility |
| Oils/Sealants | Reduce moisture loss | Jojoba Oil, Argan Oil, Grapeseed Oil | N/A | Seals moisture |
| Humectants | Attract moisture | Glycerin, Propylene Glycol | 5–8 | Increase hydration |

# CHEMICAL SERVICE CHEMISTRY

| CHEMICAL SERVICE CHEMISTRY | | | | |
|---|---|---|---|---|
| Product Type | Purpose | Common Active Ingredients | pH | Effect on Hair |
| Relaxers | Permanently straighten | Sodium Hydroxide, Calcium Hydroxide | 10–14 | Break disulfide bonds |
| No-Lye Relaxers | Texture reduction | Guanidine Hydroxide | 9–13 | Alters curl structure |
| Lighteners | Remove pigment | Ammonium Persulfate, Hydrogen Peroxide | 9–11 | Oxidize melanin |
| Permanent Color | Lift/deposit color | Ammonia, MEA, Peroxide | 8–10 | Swells cuticle |
| Demi-Permanent Color | Deposit-only color | MEA, Low-Volume Peroxide, Direct Dyes | 6–7 | Minimal cuticle disruption |

# HEAT & STYLING CHEMISTRY

**CHEMICAL SERVICE CHEMISTRY**

| Product Type | Purpose | Common Active Ingredients | pH | Effect on Hair |
|---|---|---|---|---|
| Heat Protectants | Reduce thermal stress | Dimethicone, Amodimethicone | 4–7 | Protect cuticle |
| Styling Gels | Hold curl pattern | PVP, VP/VA Copolymer | 5–8 | Forms cast around strands |
| Mousses/Foams | Lightweight hold | Polyquaternium-11, VP/VA Copolymer, Panthenol | 5–7 | Adds definition |
| Silicones | Increase shine/slip | Dimethicone, Cyclopentasiloxane, Amodimethicone | 4–7 | Smooth surface |

Scalp Spatial Distribution ™

# SSD Mapping

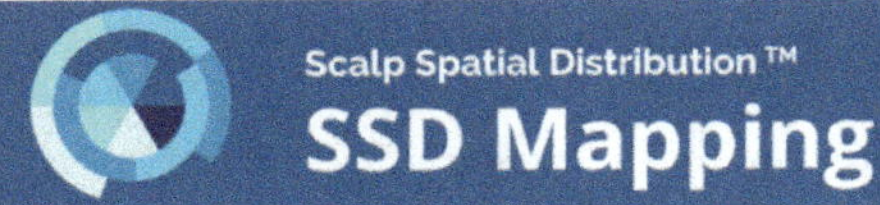

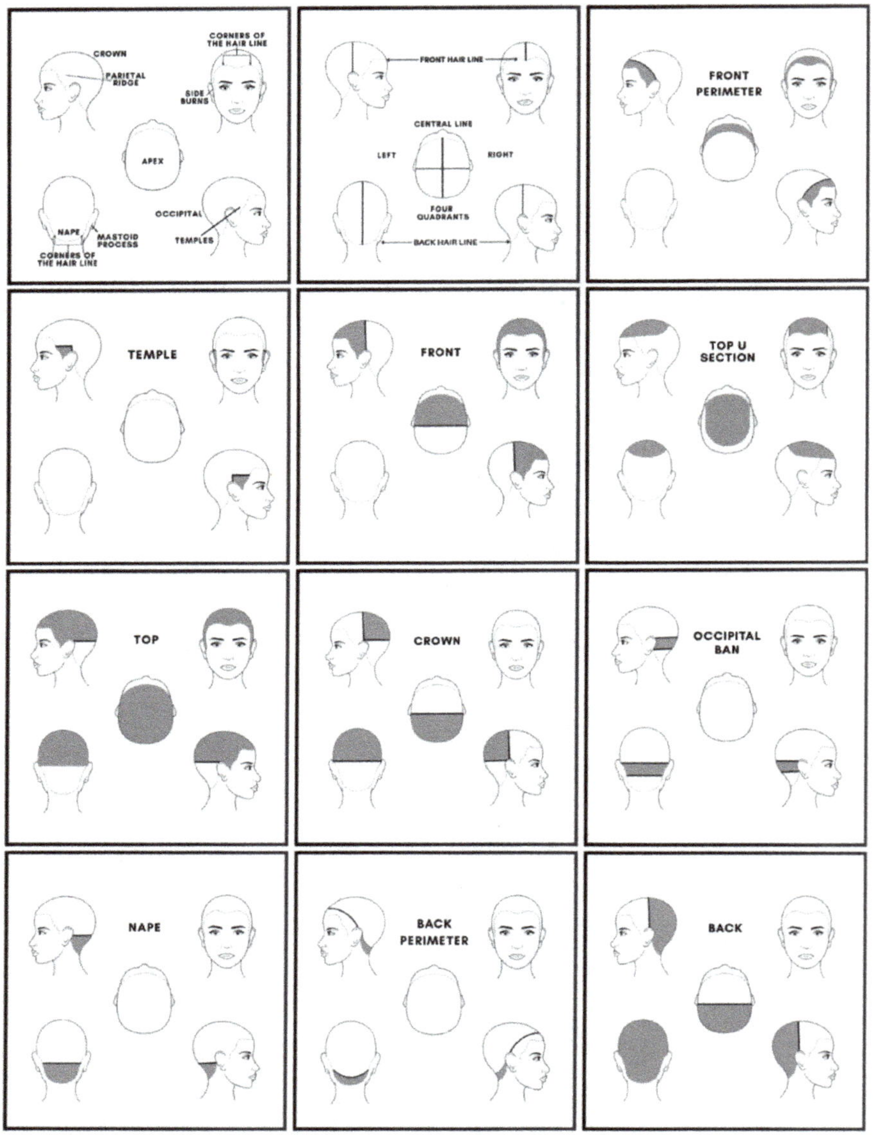
CROWN
PARIETAL RIDGE
CORNERS OF THE HAIR LINE
SIDE BURNS
APEX
NAPE
MASTOID PROCESS
CORNERS OF THE HAIR LINE
OCCIPITAL
TEMPLES
FRONT HAIR LINE
CENTRAL LINE
LEFT
RIGHT
FOUR QUADRANTS
BACK HAIR LINE
FRONT PERIMETER
TEMPLE
FRONT
TOP U SECTION
TOP
CROWN
OCCIPITAL BAN
NAPE
BACK PERIMETER
BACK

Scalp Spatial Distribution ™

# SSD Service Plan

**GUEST** ______________________ **Date** __________

**STYLIST** ______________________

**Client History:** ______________________

______________________

______________________

**Service Type:** ______________________

**Cut:** ______________________

**Color:** ______________________

**Treatment:** ______________________

______________________

**Scalp Condition:** ______________________

**Life Style:** ______________________

| Zone Service Goals | Beauty Astethics |
| --- | --- |
| | |

| Service Type | Technical Strategy |
| --- | --- |
| | |

**Product Plan:** ______________________

______________________

______________________

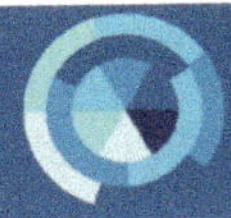

Scalp Spatial Distribution ™

# SSD MAPPING - Service Goals by Region

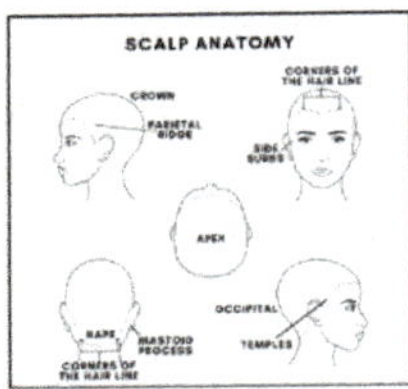


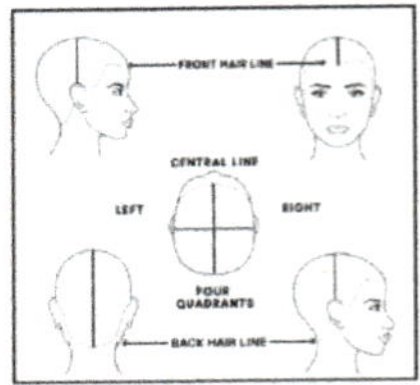

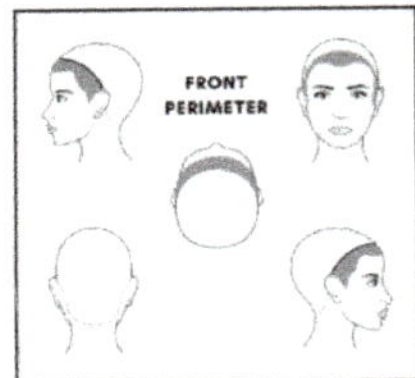


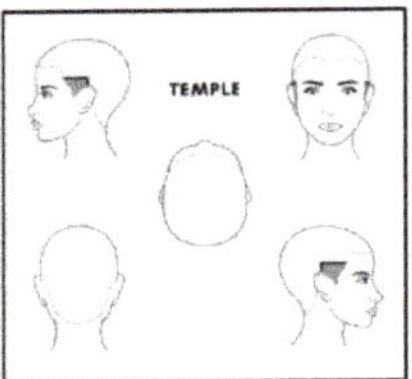


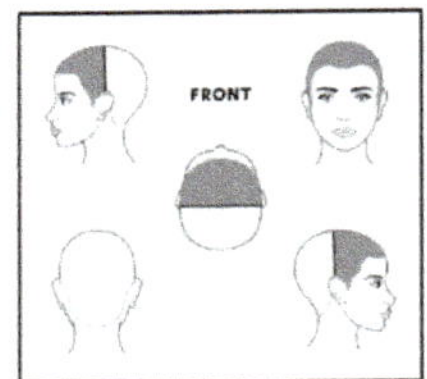


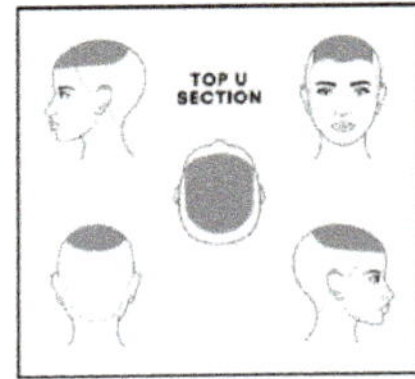


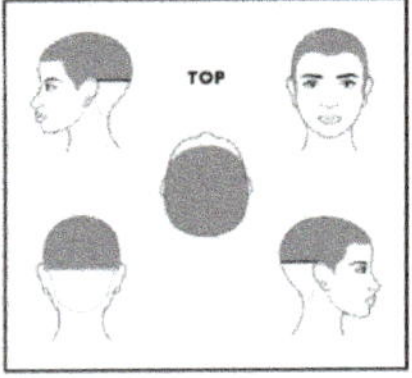


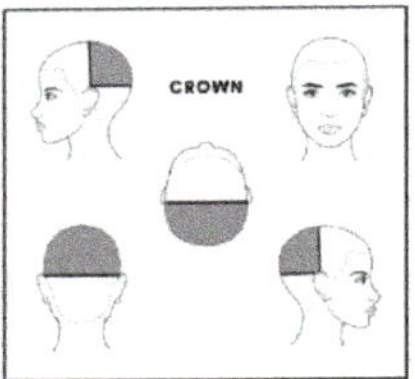


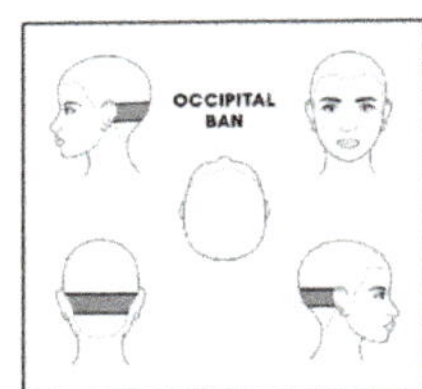


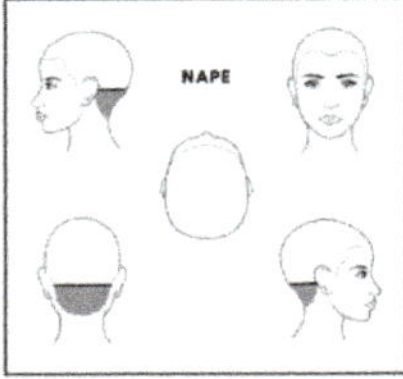


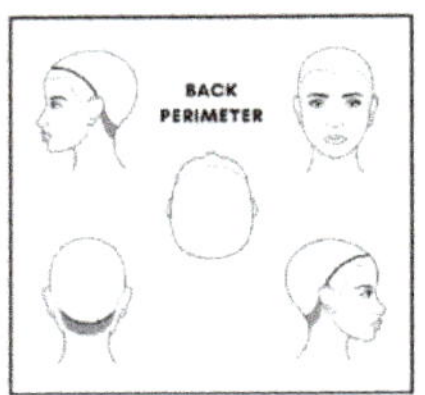


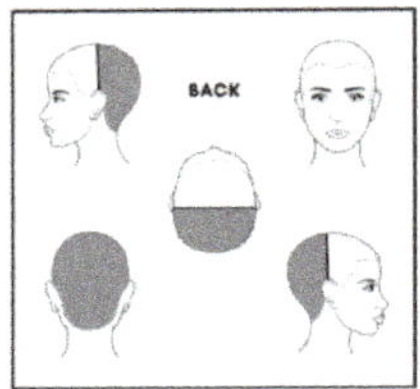

# REFERENCE

African American Museum of Iowa. "History of Hair." Accessed April 2026. https://blackiowa.org/digital-resources/utrdigitalexhibit/history-of-hair/.

African American Registry. "Black Hair Care and Its Culture, a Story." Accessed April 2026. https://aaregistry.org/story/black-hair-care-and-culture-a-story/.

African American Registry. "Annie Malone, Businesswoman Born." Accessed April 2026. https://aaregistry.org/story/annie-malone-businesswoman-original/.

"Black History and the Hot Comb, a Story." *African American Registry*, https://aaregistry.org/story/black-history-and-the-hot-comb-a-story/.

Bundles, A'Lelia. *On Her Own Ground: The Life and Times of Madam C.J. Walker*. Scribner, 2001.

Byrd, Ayana D. and Lori L. Tharps. *Hair Story: Untangling the Roots of Black Hair in America*. St. Martin's Press, 2001.

*GovDocs. "CROWN Act — States with Hair Discrimination Laws." Last modified July 2025. https://www.govdocs.com/states-with-hair-discrimination-laws/.*

*Wrapaloc Products Inc. "Hair-Story: Facts About the Bronner Brothers." February 14, 2023. https://wrapaloc.com/blogs/news/hair-story-facts-about-the-bronner-brothers.*

Rooks, Noliwe M. *Hair Raising: Beauty, Culture, and African American Women*. Rutgers University Press, 1996.

Evans, Harold, Gail Buckland, and David Lefer. *They Made America*. Little, Brown, 2004.

Nessler, Charles. *The Story of Hair.* New York: Boni and Liveright, 1928

Bedi, Joyce. "Germany | Charles (Karl) Nessler." *Invention & Technology Magazine*, 3 June 2021, https://invention.si.edu.

Walker, Andre, and Teresa Wiltz. *Andre Talks Hair!*. Simon & Schuster, 1997.

Kavitha, S., Natarajan, K., Thilagavathi, G., & Srinivas, C. R. (2016). *Effect of oil application, age, diet, and pigmentation on the tensile strength and breaking point of hair.* International Journal of Trichology, 8(4), 155–159. https://doi.org/10.4103/0974-7753.203170

Gavazzoni Dias, Maria Fernanda Reis1,2,. Hair Cosmetics: An Overview. International Journal of Trichology 7(1):p 2-15, Jan–Mar 2015. | DOI: 10.4103/0974-7753.153450

Yang F, Zhang Y, Rheinstädter MC. 2014. The structure of people's hair. *PeerJ* 2:e619 https://doi.org/10.7717/peerj.619

Milady Standard Cosmetology in APA format, you would write: Milady. (2025). *Milady Standard Cosmetology* (14th ed.). Cengage Learning.

www.ingramcontent.com/pod-product-compliance
Lightning Source LLC
LaVergne TN
LVHW081324110826
845149LV00007B/1581

* 9 7 9 8 9 9 2 5 6 6 2 2 2 *